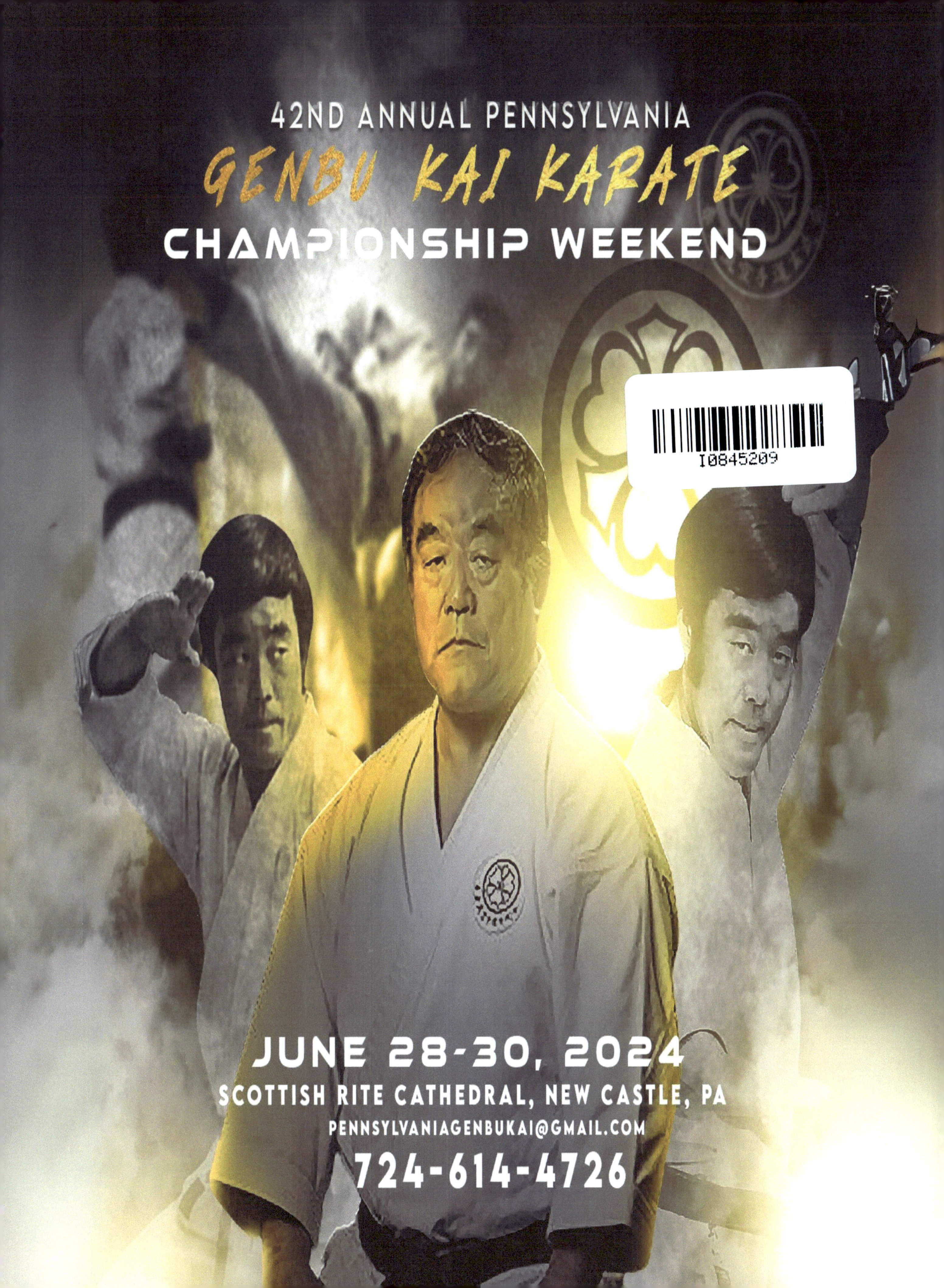

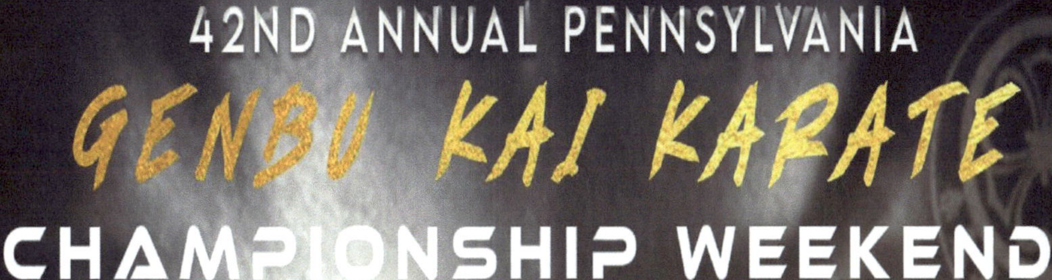
42ND ANNUAL PENNSYLVANIA
GENBU KAI KARATE
CHAMPIONSHIP WEEKEND
JUNE 28-30, 2024
SCOTTISH RITE CATHEDRAL, NEW CASTLE, PA
PENNSYLVANIAGENBUKAI@GMAIL.COM
724-614-4726

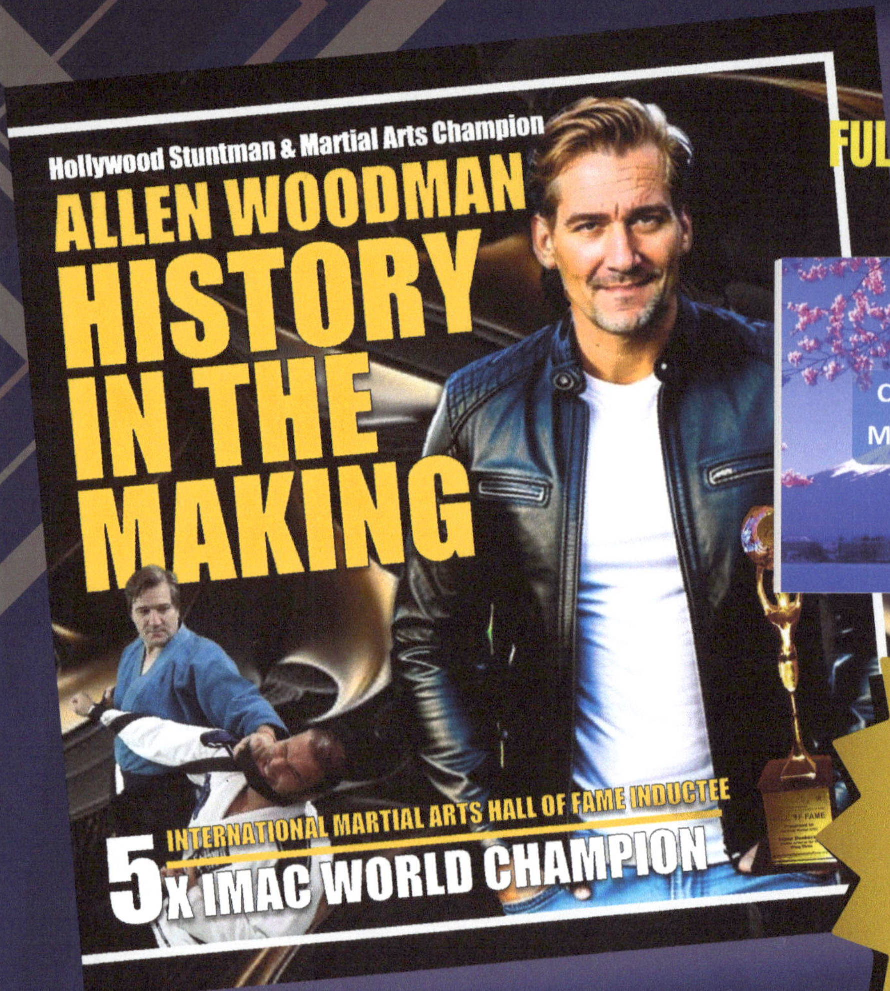

FULL COVER THROUGHOUT THE ENTIRE BOOK

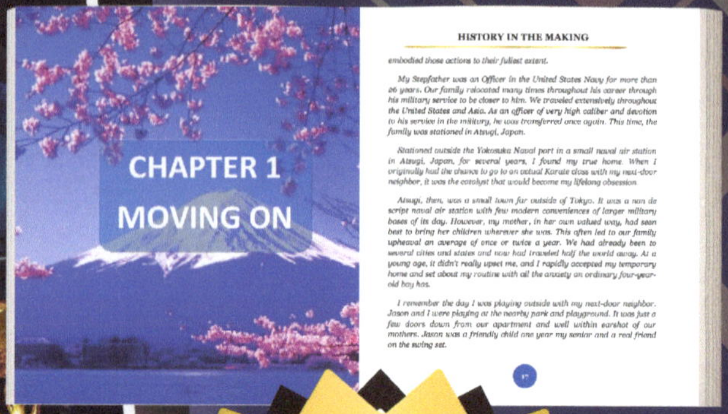

HISTORY IN THE MAKING

embodied those actions to their fullest extent.

My Stepfather was an Officer in the United States Navy for more than 26 years. Our family relocated many times throughout his career through his military service to be closer to him. We traveled extensively throughout the United States and Asia. As an officer of very high caliber and devotion to his service in the military, he was transferred once again. This time, the family was stationed in Atsugi, Japan.

Stationed outside the Yokosuka Naval port in a small naval air station in Atsugi, Japan, for several years, I found my true home. When I originally had the chance to go to an actual Karate class with my next-door neighbor, it was the catalyst that would become my lifelong obsession.

Atsugi, then, was a small town far outside of Tokyo. It was a non de script naval air station with few modern conveniences of larger military bases of its day. However, my mother, in her own valued way, had seen best to bring her children wherever she was. This often led to our family upheaval an average of once or twice a year. We had already been to several cities and states and now had traveled half the world away. At a young age, it didn't really upset me, and I rapidly accepted my temporary home and set about my routine with all the anxiety an ordinary four-year-old boy has.

I remember the day I was playing outside with my next-door neighbor. Jason and I were playing at the nearby park and playground. It was just a few doors down from our apartment and well within earshot of our mothers. Jason was a friendly child one year my senior and a real friend on the swing set.

AVAILABLE NOW $19.95

Allen Woodman has spent his entire life dedicated to martial arts, performing daring stunts, and embarking on thrilling adventures.

From a young age, Allen showed exceptional talent in martial arts. He trained tirelessly, honing his skills and becoming a champion in various disciplines. His passion for adventure led him to travel to different countries, immersing himself in different cultures and learning from the best martial artists around the world. But Allen's story isn't just about martial arts.

With a keen business mind. He successfully established several businesses in different countries, making a name for himself as an entrepreneur. His ability to adapt to new environments and connect with people from different backgrounds played a crucial role in his success.

Throughout his journey, Allen encountered numerous challenges and obstacles. But he faced them with determination and a positive outlook. His wit and perspective on life makes him a captivating storyteller, sharing his incredible journey with the world. In his book, Allen recounts his 50 years of life experiences. His unique perspective on life, adventure, and business made his story a captivating read for anyone seeking inspiration and excitement.

His story serves as a reminder that with dedication, resilience, and a positive mindset, anyone can overcome challenges and create a life filled with adventure, success, and fulfillment. If you're looking for a captivating story that combines martial arts, adventure, and business, Allen Woodman's book is a must-read. Prepare to be inspired, entertained, and motivated.

$4.95 FULL COLOR DIGITAL VERSION ONLINE WWW.ISSUU.COM

AVAILABLE ON AMAZON.COM

TABLE OF
Contents

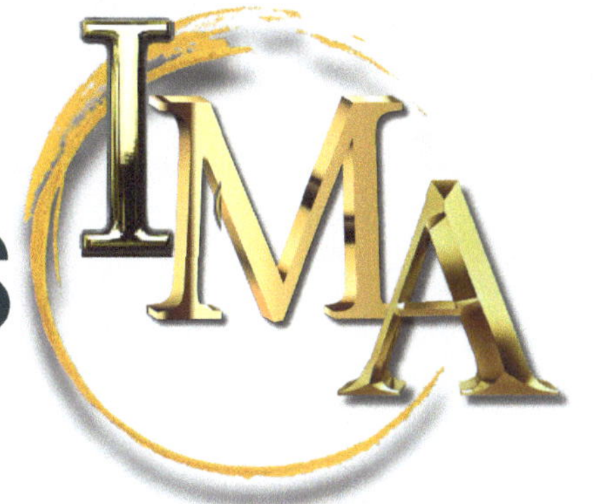

INTERNATIONAL MARTIAL ARTS MAGAZINE

BIG SALE

GET UP TO 30% OFF

APPLY DIRECLY FOR A FULL YEAR SUBSCRIPTION

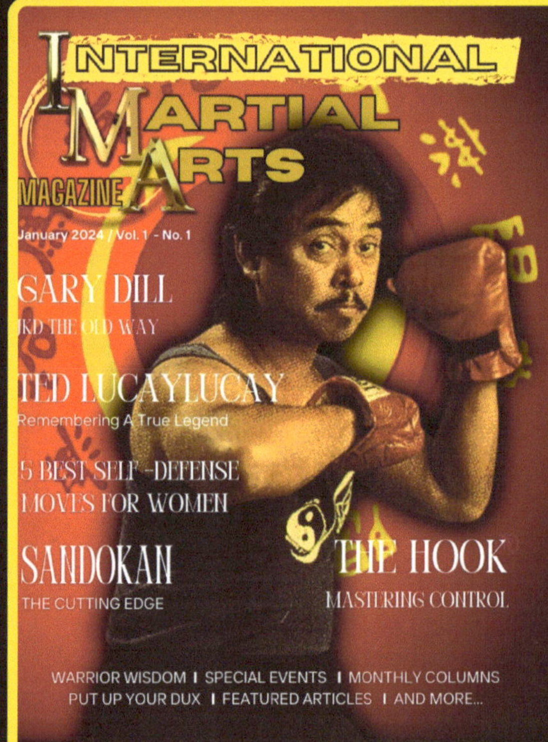

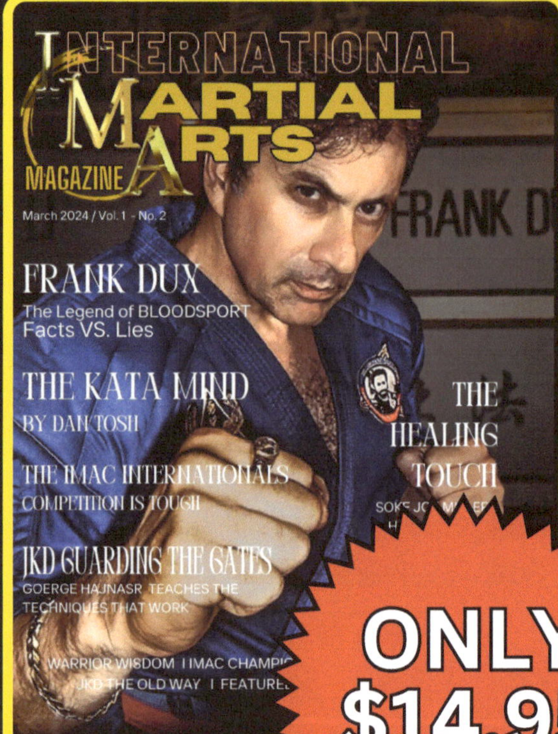

ONLY $14.95 Per Issue

BI MONTHLY INDUSTRY MAGAZINE

International Martial Arts Magazine is a NEW Bi-Monthly magazine focused on all the various aspects of martial arts. With fascinating and riveting articles and featured stories along with columnists like the martial arts ICON Frank Dux of "Bloodsport" fame, Author Bohdi Sanders, Legendary instructor Gary Dill, and many more. Join us each month as we bring you all the excitement and information on the martial arts world around you. From traditional martial arts to new progressive theories and practices, this magazine allows you an inside look at the arts and the people that make them great.
Join us for each issue.

Contact us directly to apply for a yearly subscription.
All orders must be paid in full to receive the annual 30% discount.

artseastpublish@gmail.com

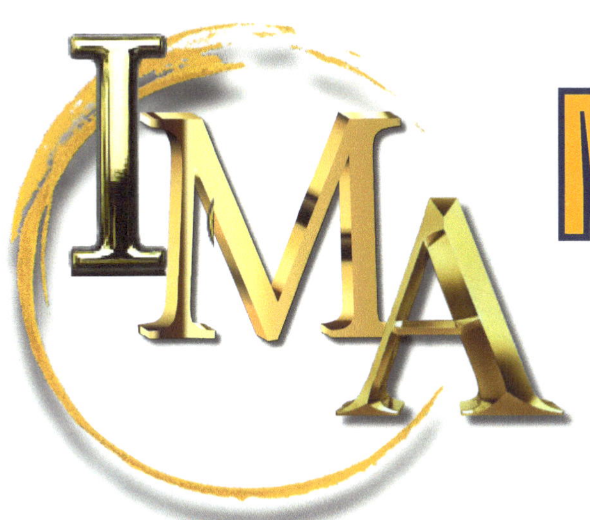

MAGAZINE

LETTER FROM THE EDITOR

To our readers,

I hope this message finds you well. I wanted to introduce myself as the editor-in-chief and creative designer of INTERNATIONAL MARTIAL ARTS MAGAZINE. With over 50 years of hands-on experience in multiple martial arts, I have dedicated my life to training and understanding martial arts practice and self-defense.

Throughout my journey, I have had the privilege of training with some of history's most amazing masters and instructors. This unique perspective allows me to bring a fresh outlook to the theories, ideas, history, and people within the martial arts community.

While I have been honored by the martial arts history museum and inducted into several martial arts Hall of fame events, I am always looking forward and never resting on past accolades. As a competitive person, I have also had the opportunity to compete on the international stage, becoming a five-time world champion at the Internationals in Las Vegas from 2016 to 2021.

Our magazine, in its first issue this past January, has already reached over 13,000 people worldwide. We are published in 10 countries and in 8 languages, striving to be a truly multi-lingual international source of information for the entire martial arts community.

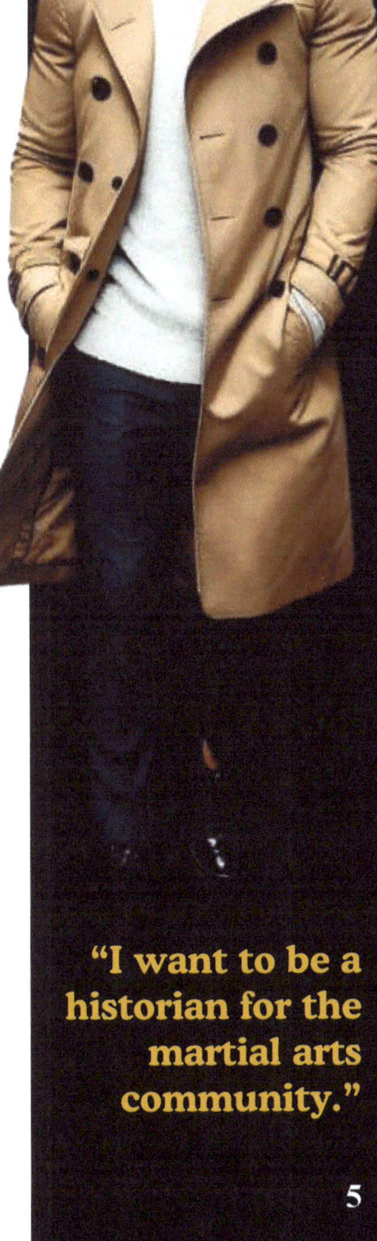

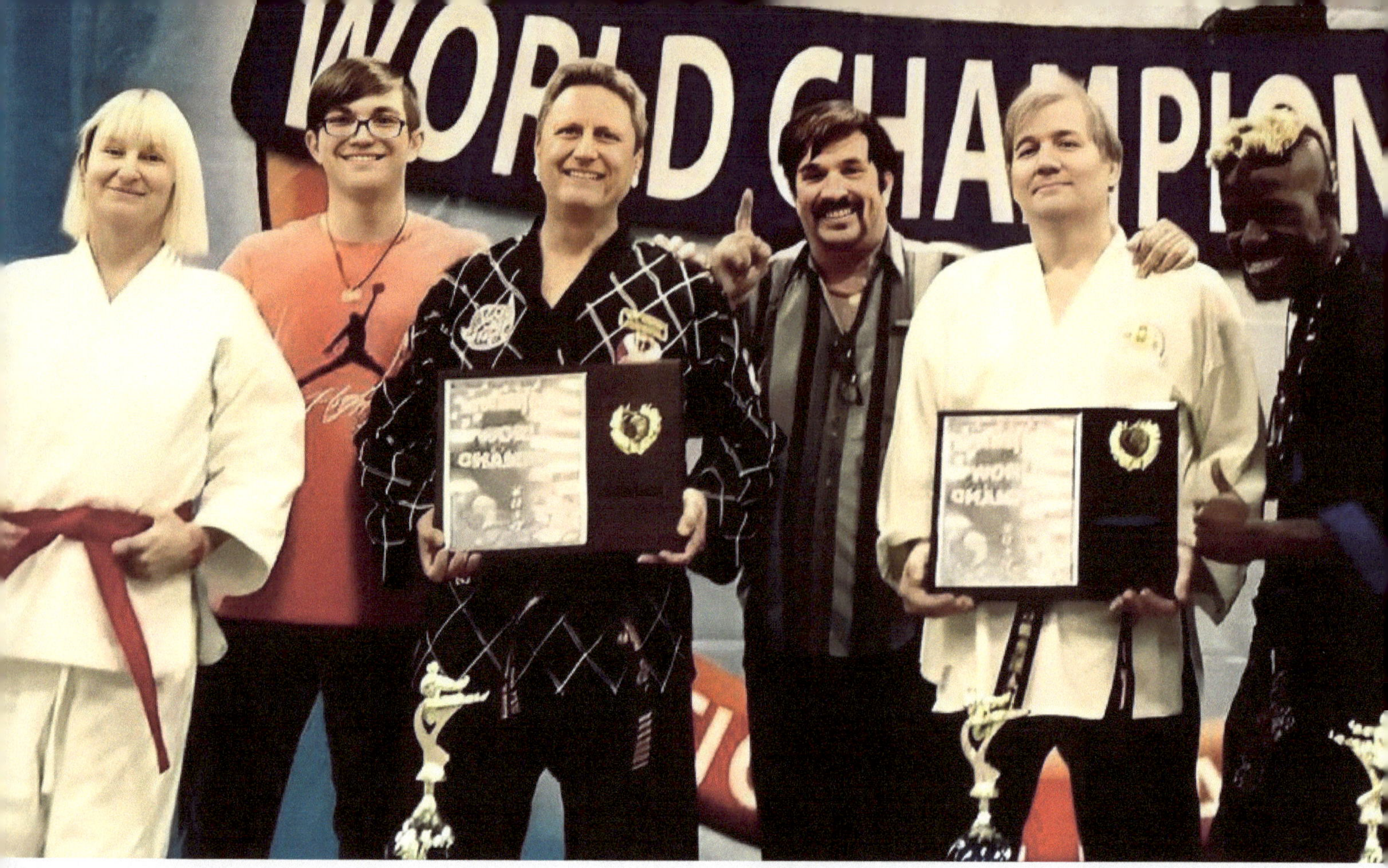

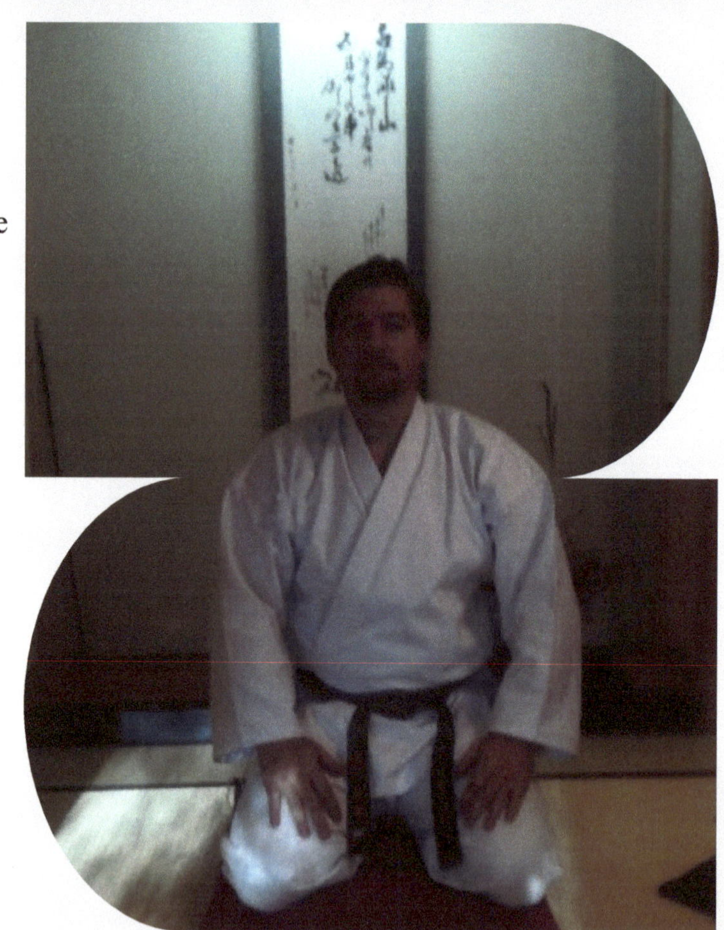

I invite you to join us in the next edition of INTERNATIONAL MARTIAL ARTS MAGAZINE. Together, we will continue to research and tell the stories of amazing arts, styles, and systems, as well as the incredible instructors and students who practice and share these arts with others.

Thank you for your support, and I look forward to your continued readership.

Allen Woodman

Best regards,
Allen Woodman
Editor-in-Chief and Creative Designer
INTERNATIONAL MARTIAL ARTS
MAGAZINE

DRAGON WEAR

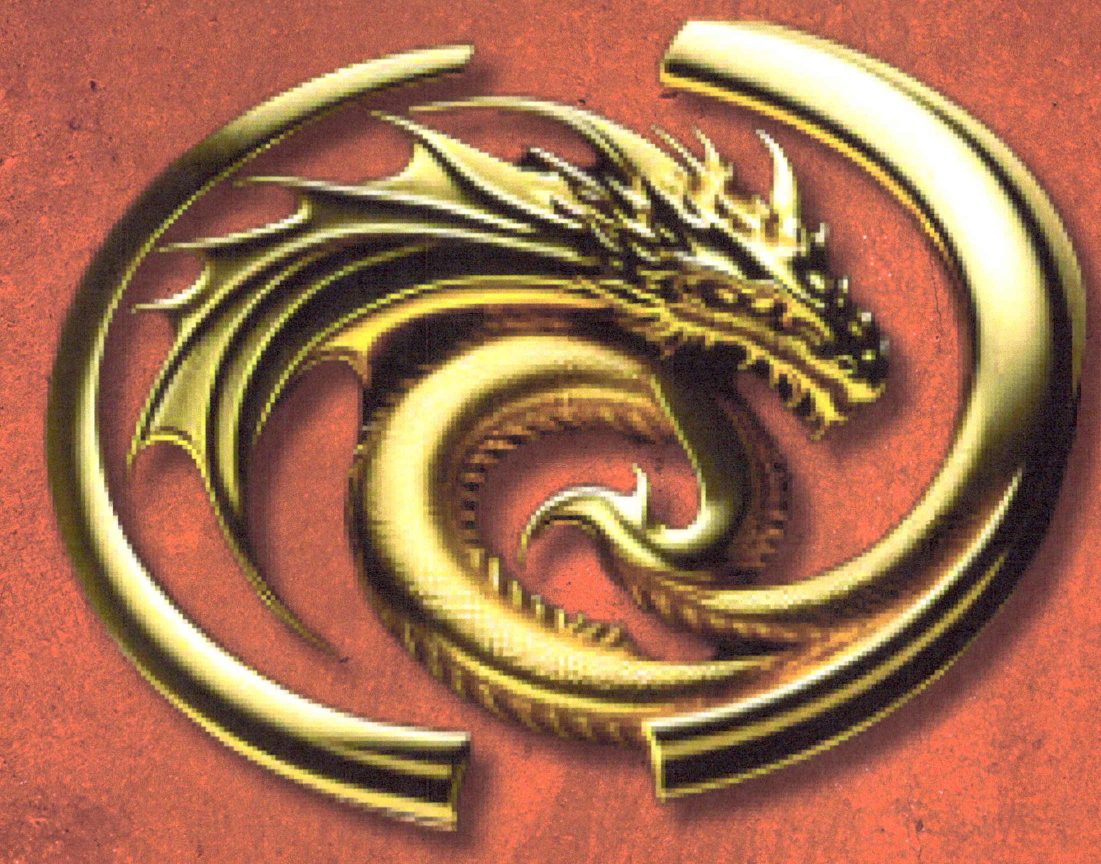

WWW.DRAGONWEARBRAND.COM

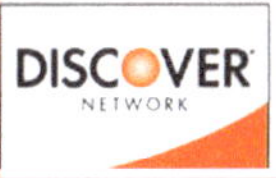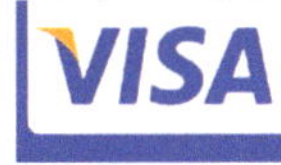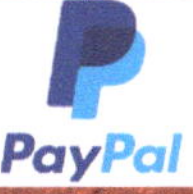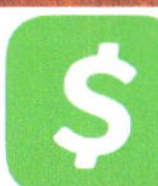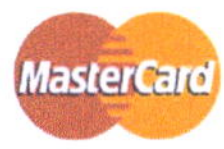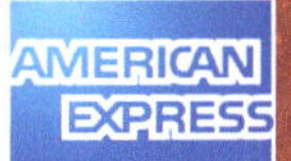

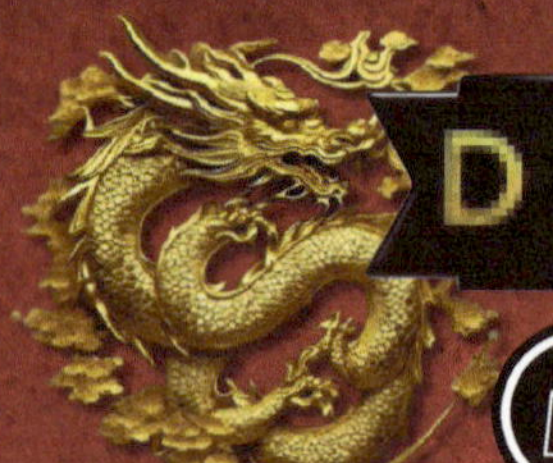
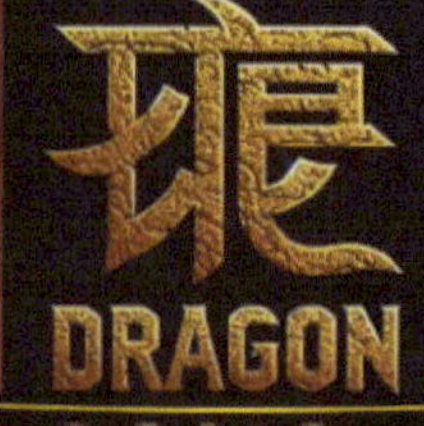
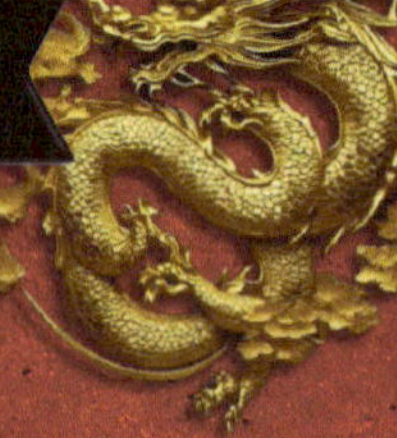

DRAGON WE·AR

SHOP NOW **BUY NOW**

1 (725) 377 - 8092   **1 (725) 377 - 8092**

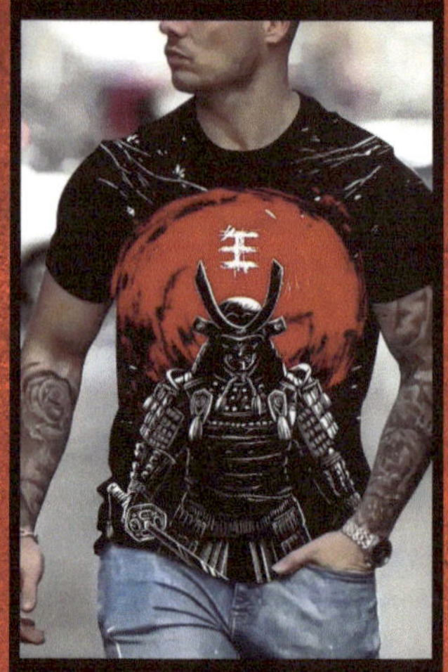
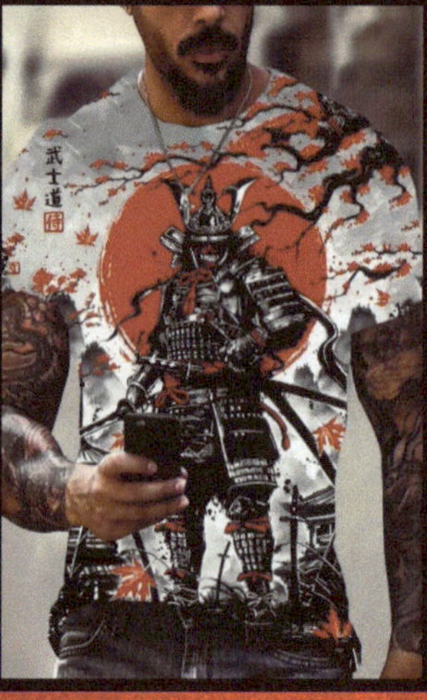

Black / Red
$19.95 + S&H

White / Blk / Red
$19.95 + S&H

Sizes S / M / L / XL / XXl

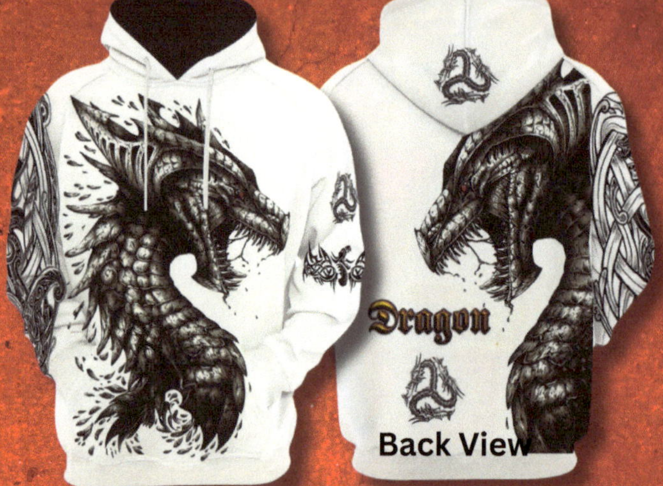
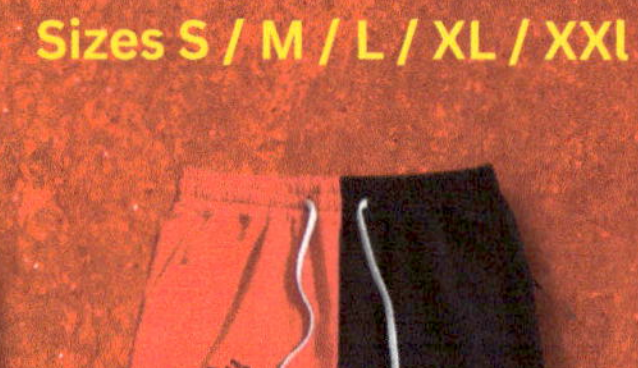

White & Blk
$19.95 + S&H

Sizes S / M / L / XL / XXl

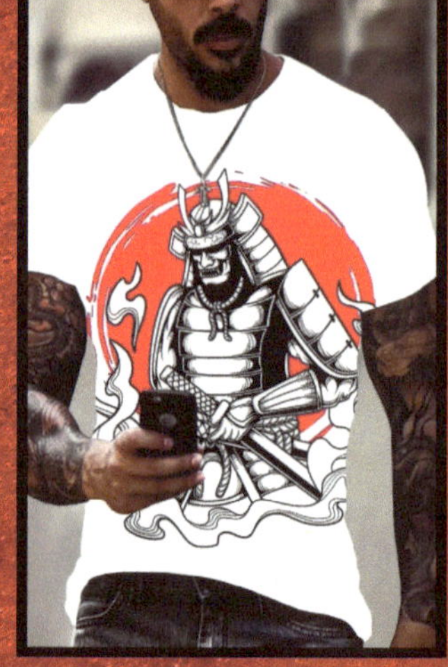
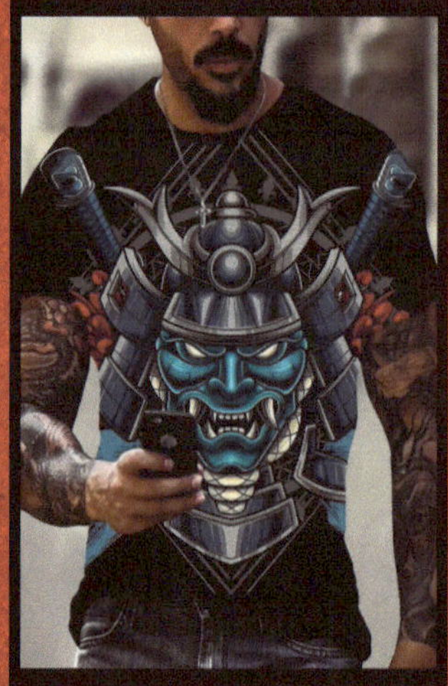
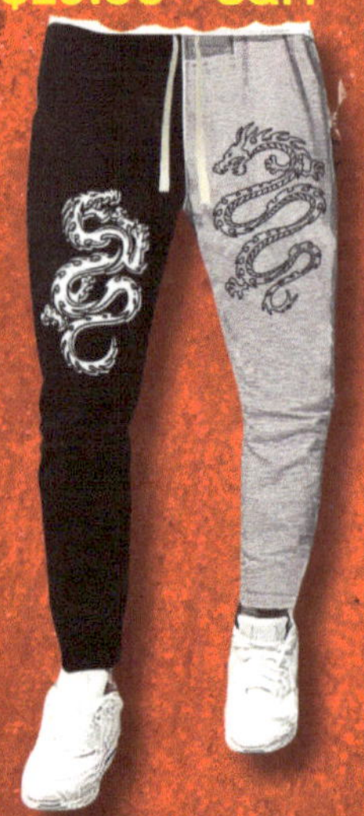
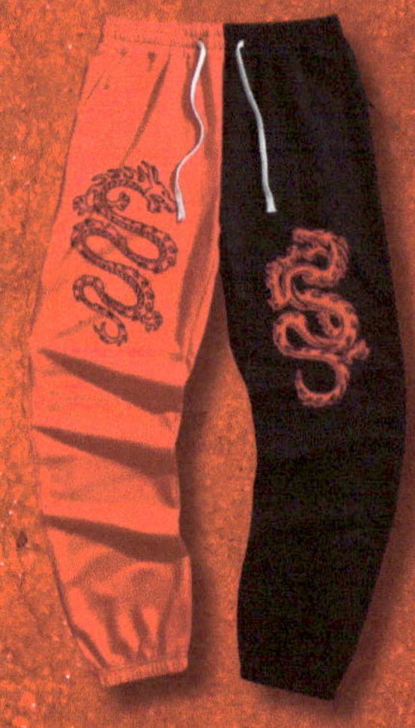

White / Red / Blk
$19.95 + S&H

Blk / Grey
$19.95 + S&H

Black & Grey
$19.95 + S&H

Black & Red
$19.95 + S&H

Sizes S / M / L / XL / XXl

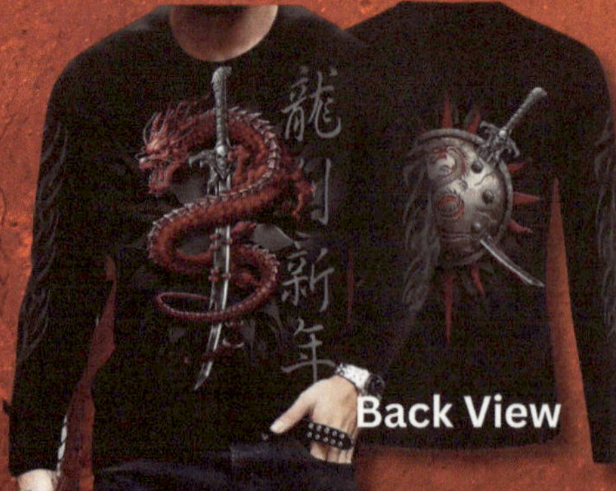

Mens
Long Sleeve
Blk / Red / Grey
$19.95 + S&H

Women's Long Sleeve
Black
Sizes 6-14.5
$19.95 + S&H

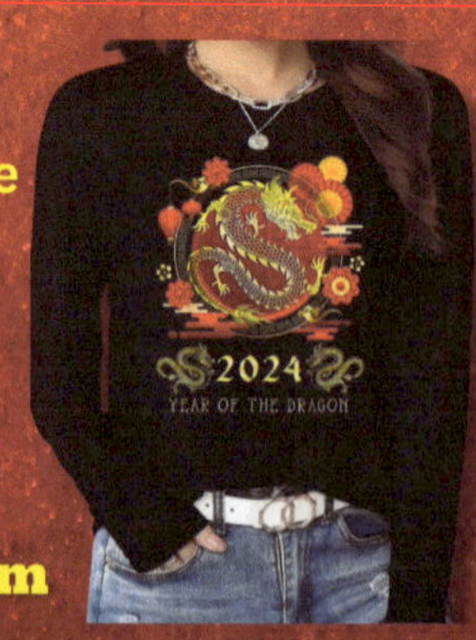

Dragonwearbranddesign@gmail.com

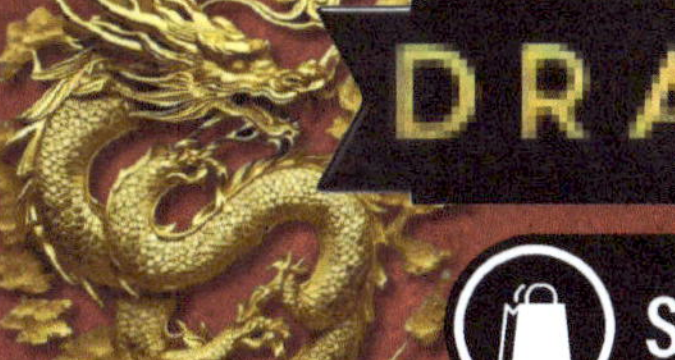
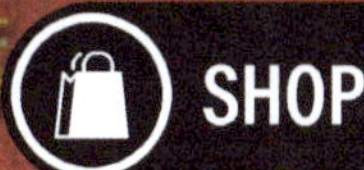
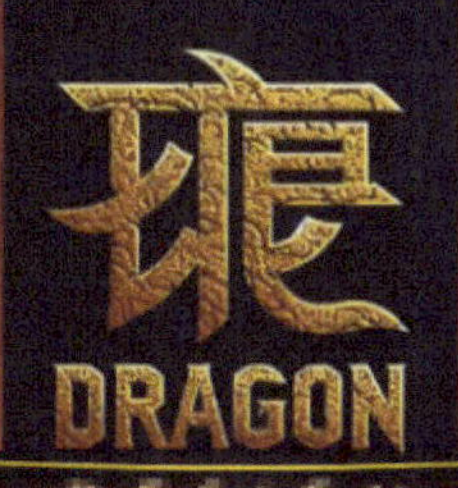
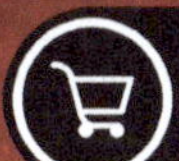
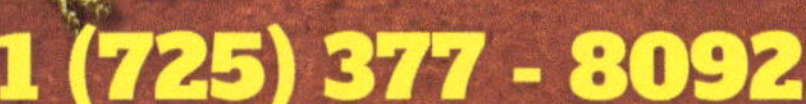

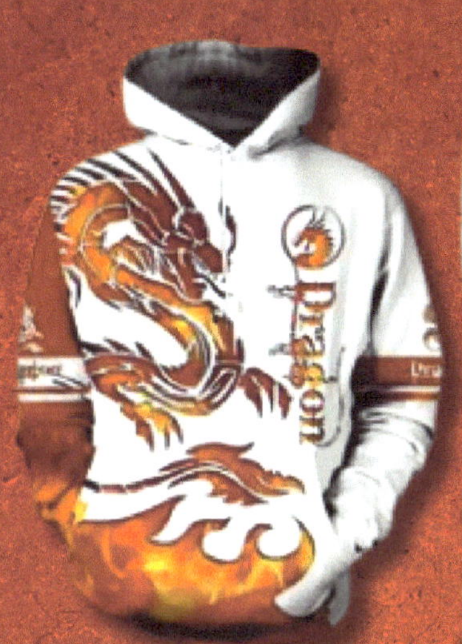

White & Orange
$39.95 + S&H

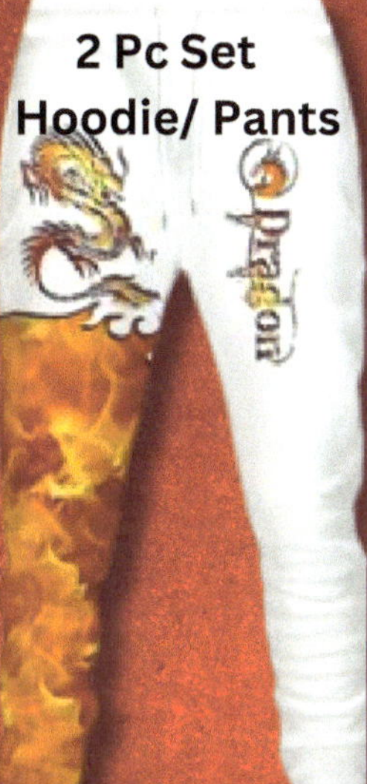

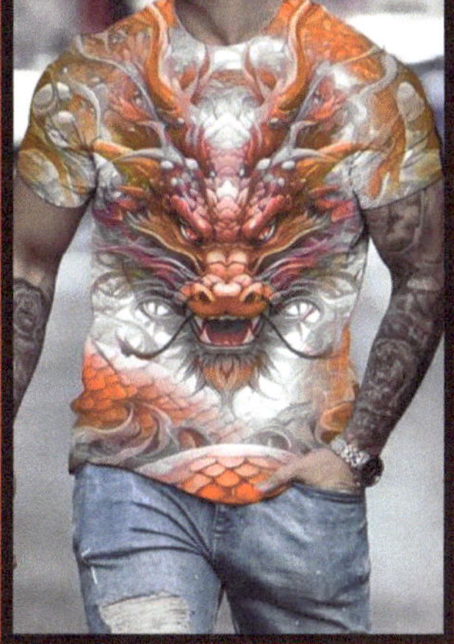

Available Colors
Mixed - Blue - Orange
$19.95 + S&H

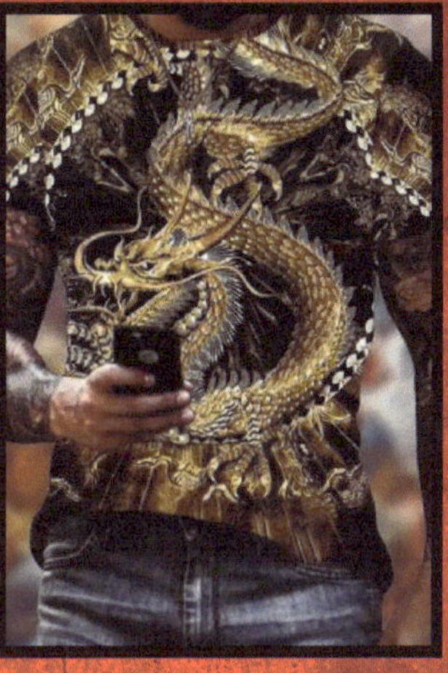

Black & Gold
$19.95 + S&H

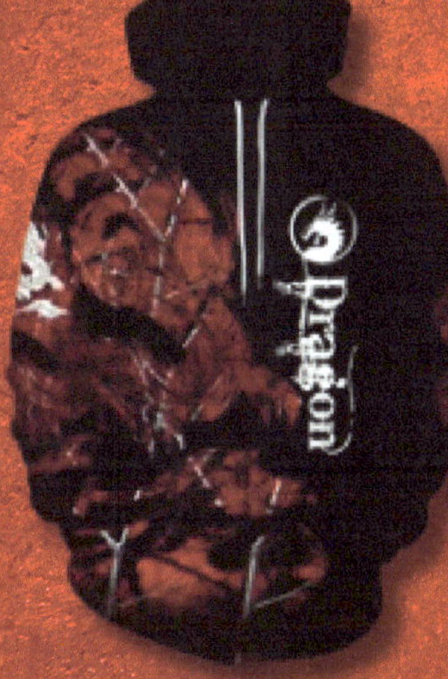

Black & Red
$39.95 + S&H

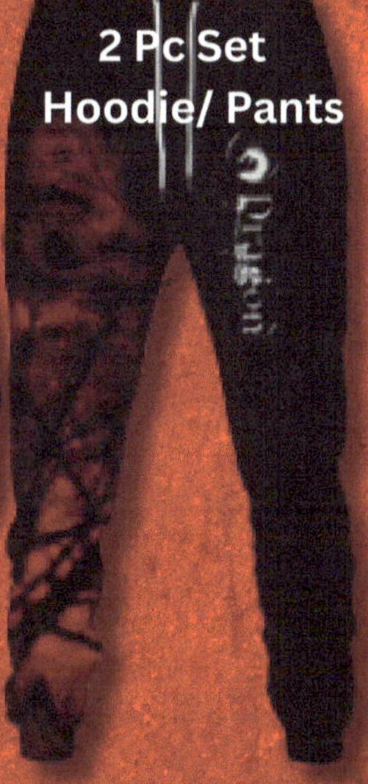

Sizes S / M / L / XL / XXl

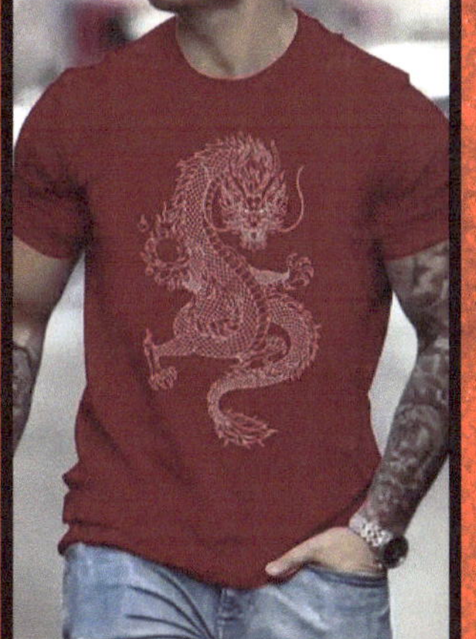

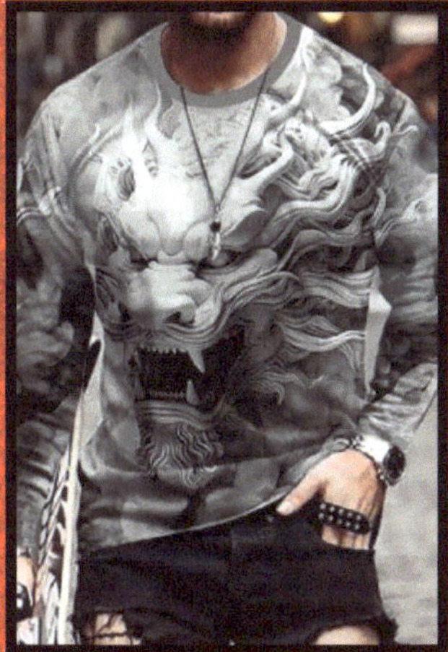

Available Colors
Blk / Sky Bl / Nvy / Grey
Drk Grn / Rd
$19.95 + S&H

Grey
$19.95 + S&H

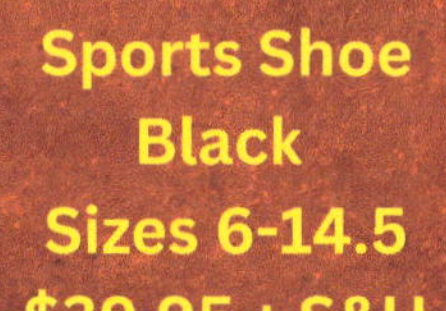

Sports Shoe
Black
Sizes 6-14.5
$39.95 + S&H

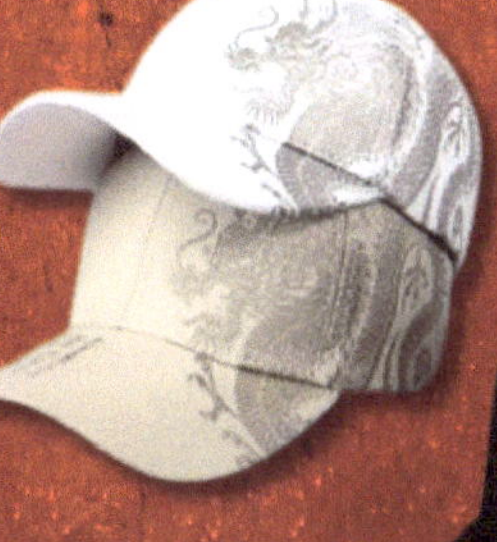

Men's Baseball Cap
Blk / Biege / Wht
$14.95 + S&H

www.dragonwearbrand.com

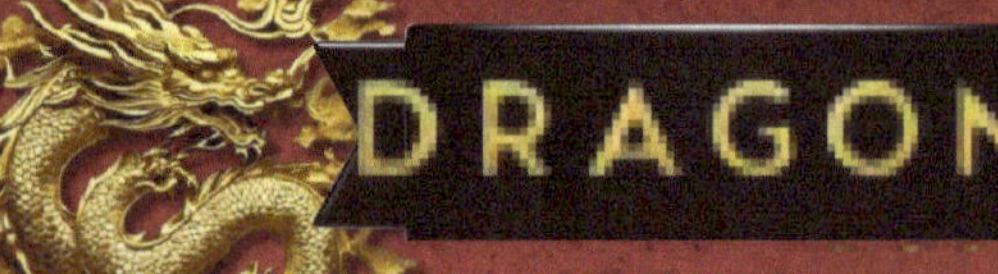
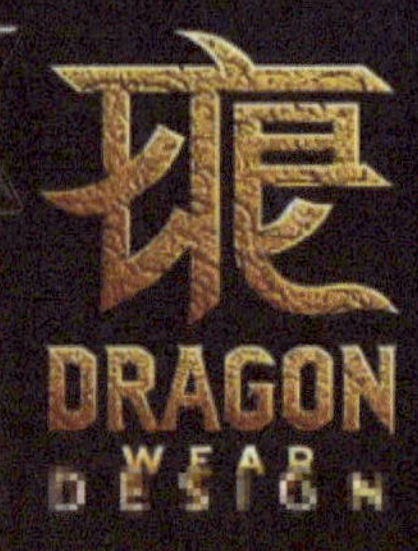

1 (725) 377 - 8092

1 (725) 377 - 8092

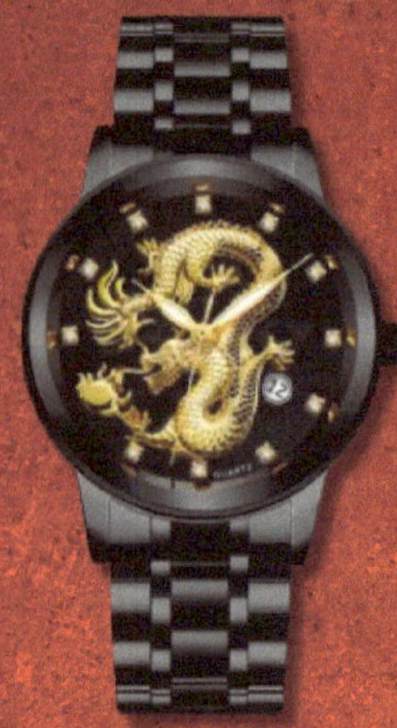

Black Watch
$25.95 + S&H

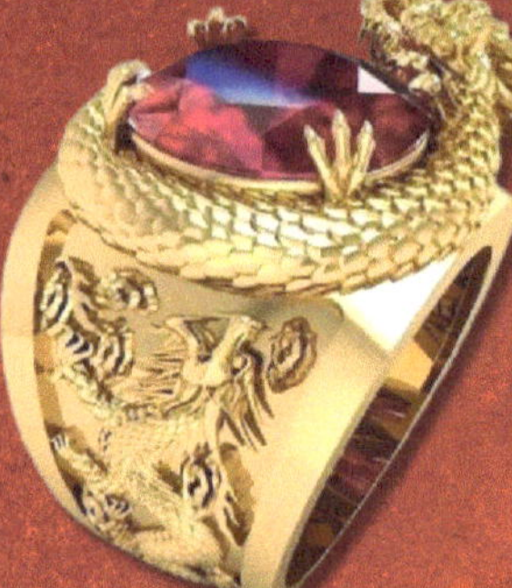

Gold Ring
$19.95 + S&H

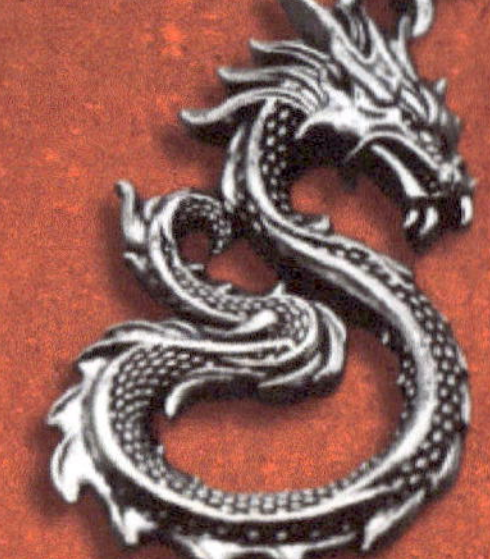

Gold Necklace
$9.95 + S&H

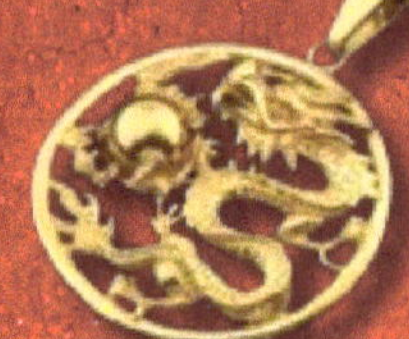

Gold Necklace
$9.95 + S&H

Silver Necklace
$9.95 + S&H

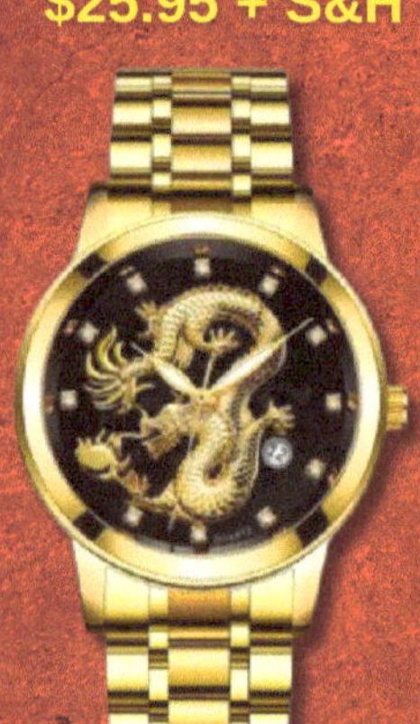

Gold / Blk
$25.95 + S&H

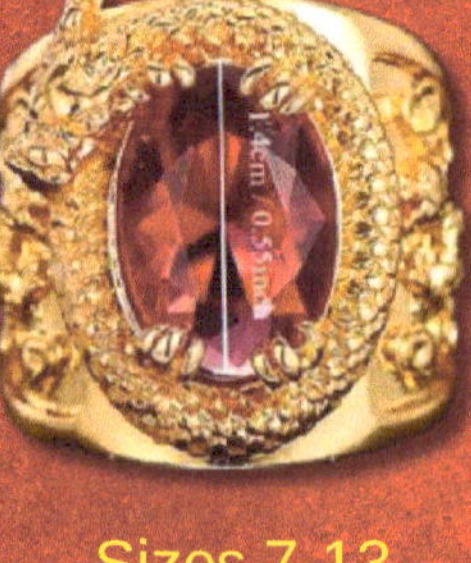

Sizes 7-13
$19.95 + S&H

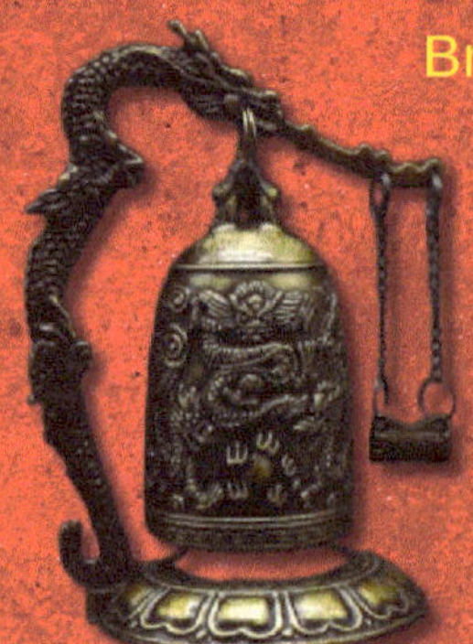

Bronze Desk Gong
6 inch X3 Inch
$19.95 + S&H

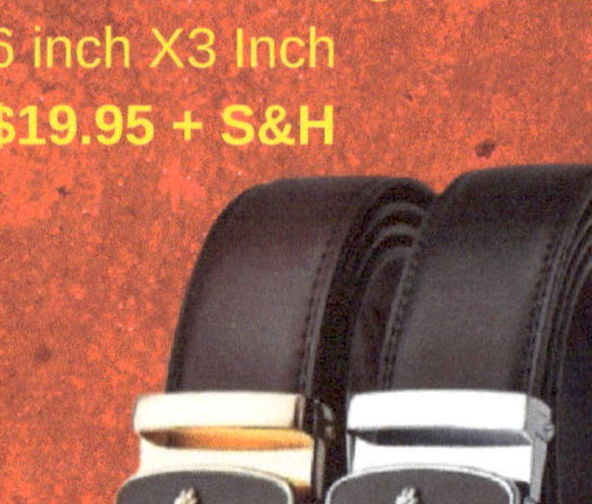

Brwn / Blk Automaitic Buckle
$19.95 + S&H

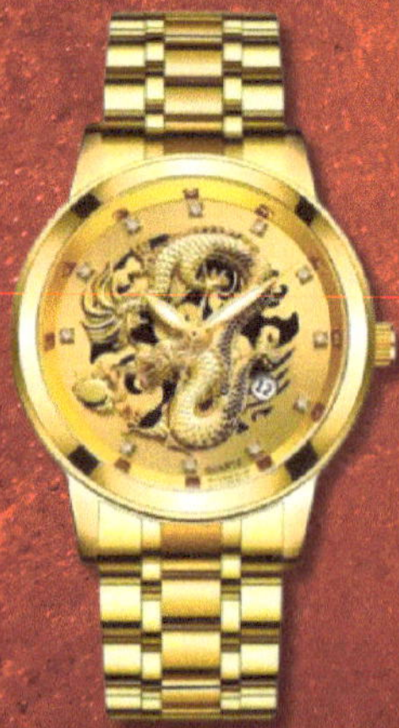

Gold / Gold
$25.95 + S&H

Gold Lapel Pin
$9.95 + S&H

Silver Lapel Pin
$9.95 + S&H

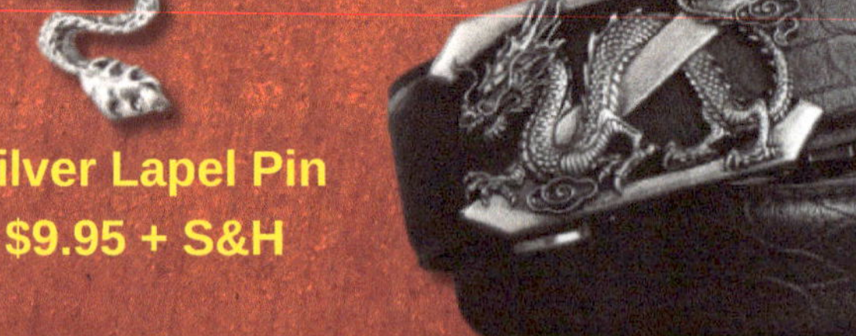

Brwn / Blk
$19.95 + S&H

www.dragonwearbrand.com

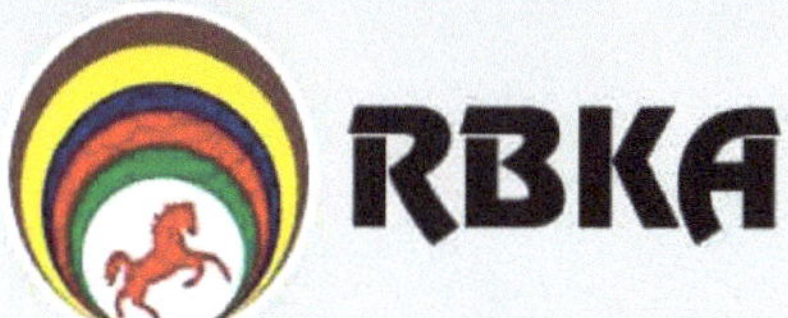

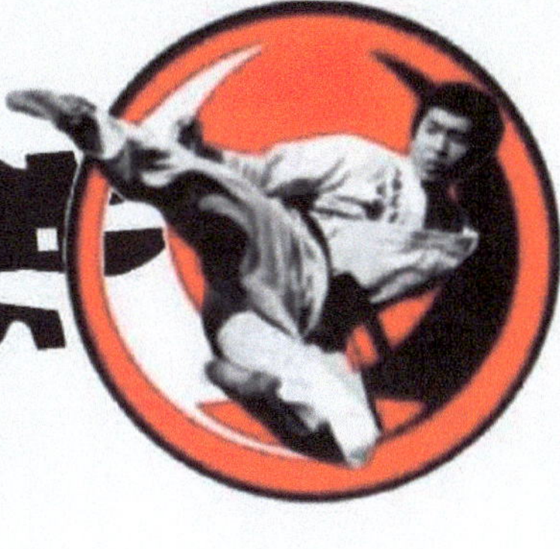

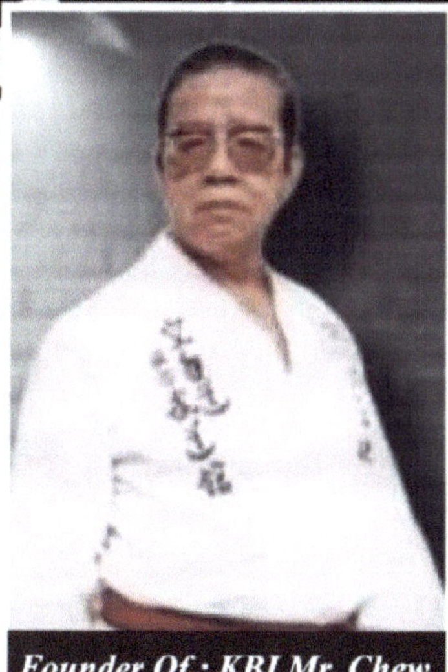
Founder Of : KBI Mr. Chew

KBI

INTERNATIONAL OPEN KARATE CHAMPIONSHIP

Date : 4th & 5th January 2025

Last Date For Registration 1st December 2024

Organised By

VASANT SHETTY
National Technical Chief of India

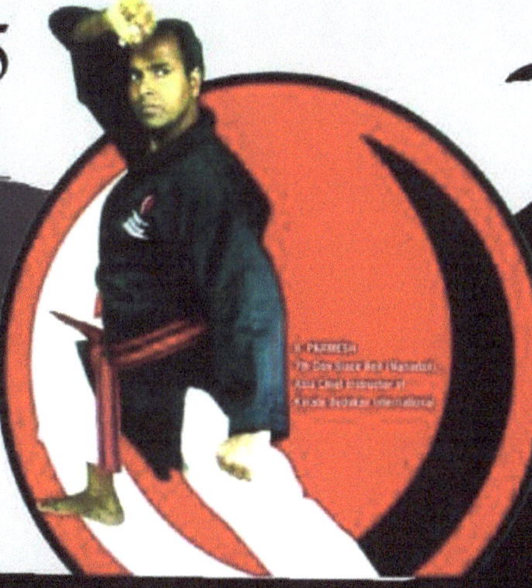
B. PARMESH
Asia Chief Instructor of KBI

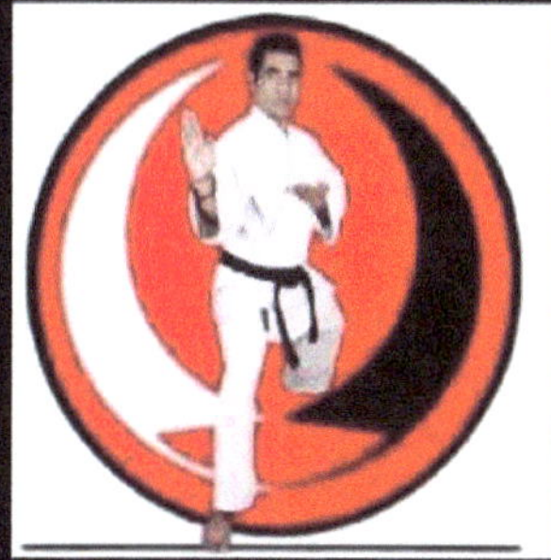
ORGANIZER
VIJAY POOJARY
9870005665

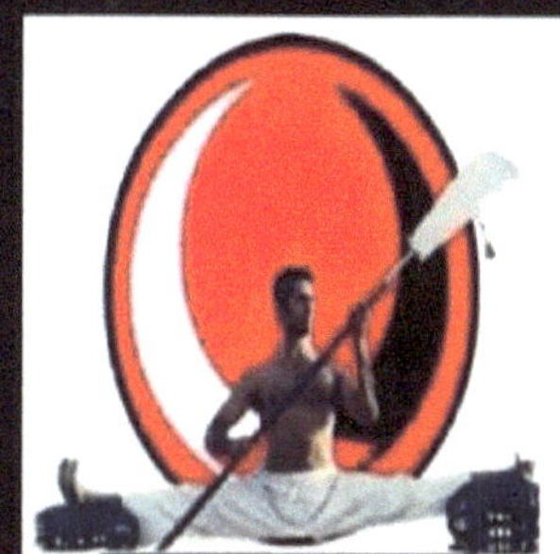
ORGANIZER
VASANT T. SHETTY
9821316584 / 9004320590

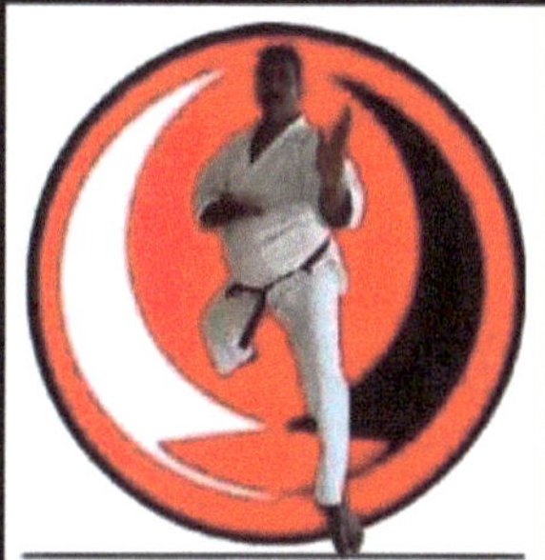
ORGANIZER
VIJAY SHETTY
7975234027

Venue : J.N.R. Kalamandir N.H. 66, Yedthare Bydoor, Dist. Udupi, Karnataka

www.vasantshettykarate.com / vasantshettykarate@yahoo.co.in

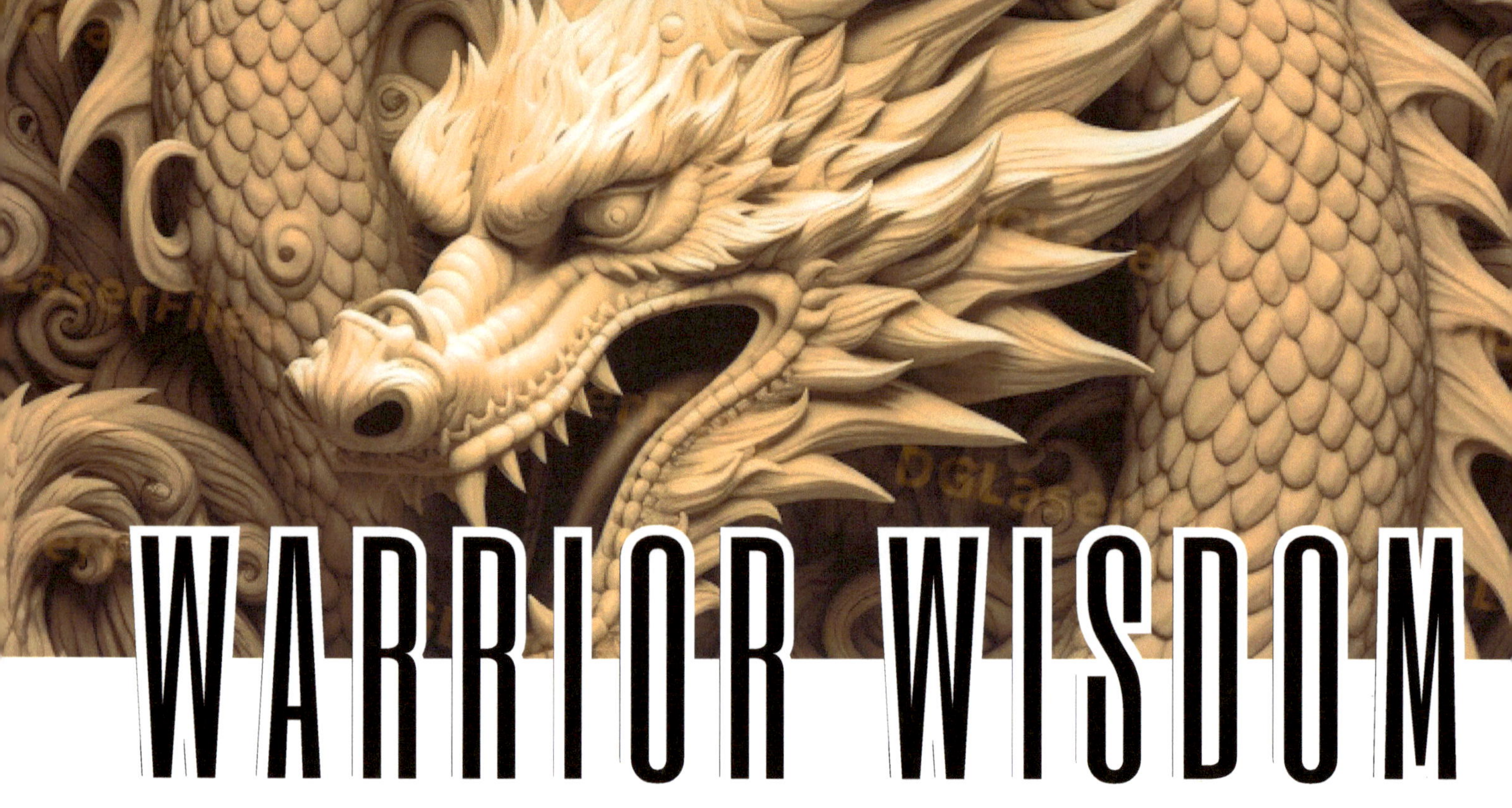

WARRIOR WISDOM

Fighting with Honor or Fighting to Survive

Bohdi Sanders, Ph.D.

Whenever I write an article about fighting, it always seems to spark a debate about whether one should fight with honor or fight to win by any means necessary. Of course, true martial artists want to live a life of honor and integrity, but where does one draw the line between living with honor and fighting with honor?

There is an easy answer to that question. Fighting with honor is only applicable in the dojo or in competition. Sparring in the dojo or in a tournament is not the same as being in a real fight. This is a point that most martial artists understand, but many are still confused about when it comes to the question of fighting with honor.

I have heard many martial artists say that one should always fight with honor, whether in training or a real fight. While this is an honorable idea, the reality of this philosophy is that it will get you badly hurt or even killed. This is primarily a philosophy held by those who have never been in a real fight.

Be that as it may, this is a debate that is centuries old. Even during the 1600s, the samurai were disgusted with Miyamoto Musashi because he refused to fight by the samurai's strict rules of engagement. They claimed that Musashi had no honor because of his tactics in his sword duels.

Musashi refused to play by the samurai's rules, instead choosing to walk away from every sword fight victoriously. He would show up late, insult his opponent, show up early to get an advantage, or even throw sand or dirt into his opponent's eyes.

The samurai considered these tactics fighting dirty and with no honor, but Musashi considered them nothing more than survival and good strategy. Did Miyamoto Musashi lack honor because he fought by his own rules? Absolutely not! The 20th principle of Musashi's Dokkodo states, "You may abandon your own body, but you must preserve your honor."

While the samurai and Musashi's other opponents were concerned about etiquette and manufactured rules, Musashi was only concerned about survival and winning by any means necessary. We all know whose philosophy led to victory and whose ideologies led to defeat.

Miyamoto Musashi understood the reality of a life-or-death fight. In a real battle, you must use anything and everything to walk away victoriously. Honor plays no part in that situation; the only thing that matters is walking away with your life intact.

An authentic martial artist fights only to protect someone else or if he has no other choice.

An honorable martial artist has no desire to use their martial arts skills to hurt another person. He has no problem walking away from an explosive situation, even if it appears to others that he is a coward.

After all, he is not concerned with the opinions of others; he is only concerned with living according to his code of honor.

"You may abandon your own body, but you must preserve your honor."

MIYAMOTO MUSASHI

When your life is on the line, there is no such thing as fighting with honor; there is only fighting to survive and walk away with as few injuries as possible. It would be best to use whatever you need to survive, whether a weapon, a brick, or throwing sand in your enemy's eyes.

That said, every true martial artist knows he or she must do everything possible to avoid a fight. Try your best to de-escalate the situation and walk away if possible.

What others think or say about his actions is meaningless.

This was obviously Musashi's attitude as well. He did not care that the samurai considered his tactics dishonorable. Like every true warrior, Musashi had a purpose behind everything he did.

He knew that if he could anger his opponent or get into his opponent's mind, the fight was pretty much over.

WARRIOR WISDOM *Cont...*

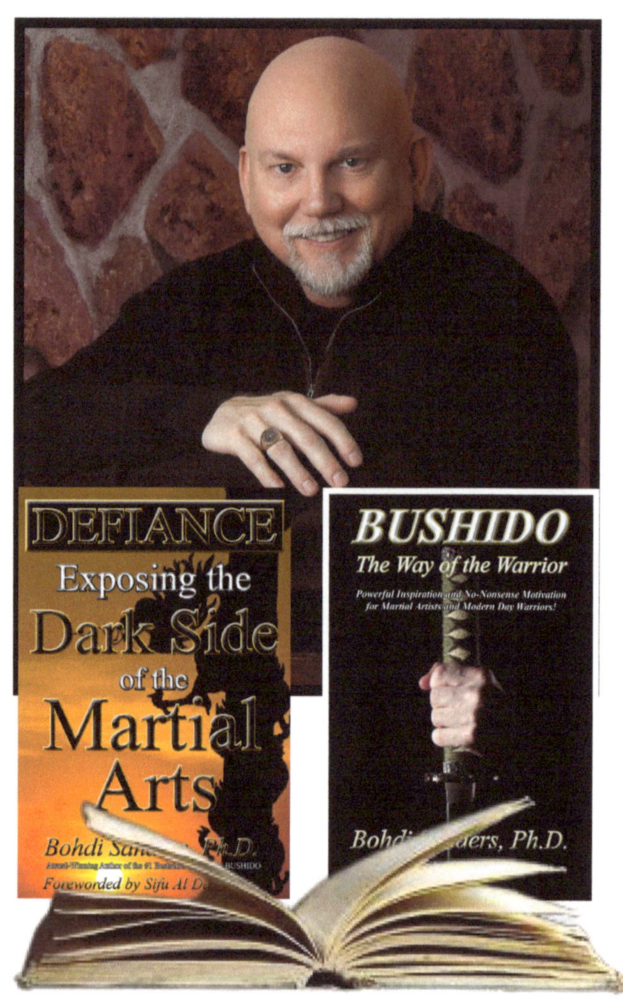

His actions were not dishonorable but rather a specific strategy to defeat his opponents.

Think about it. If you were in a fight to the death, would you be concerned about whether you survived the fight or what your opponent thought about your tactics?

The samurai were worried about saving face; Musashi was focused on survival. It is obvious who had the correct mindset in those circumstances!

Bohdi Sanders is a 5th-degree black belt in Shotokan Karate and a bestselling and award-winning author of 16 books, mainly on martial arts and warrior philosophy. Dr. Sanders' books are available on his website, www.thewisdomwarrior.com , and Amazon.

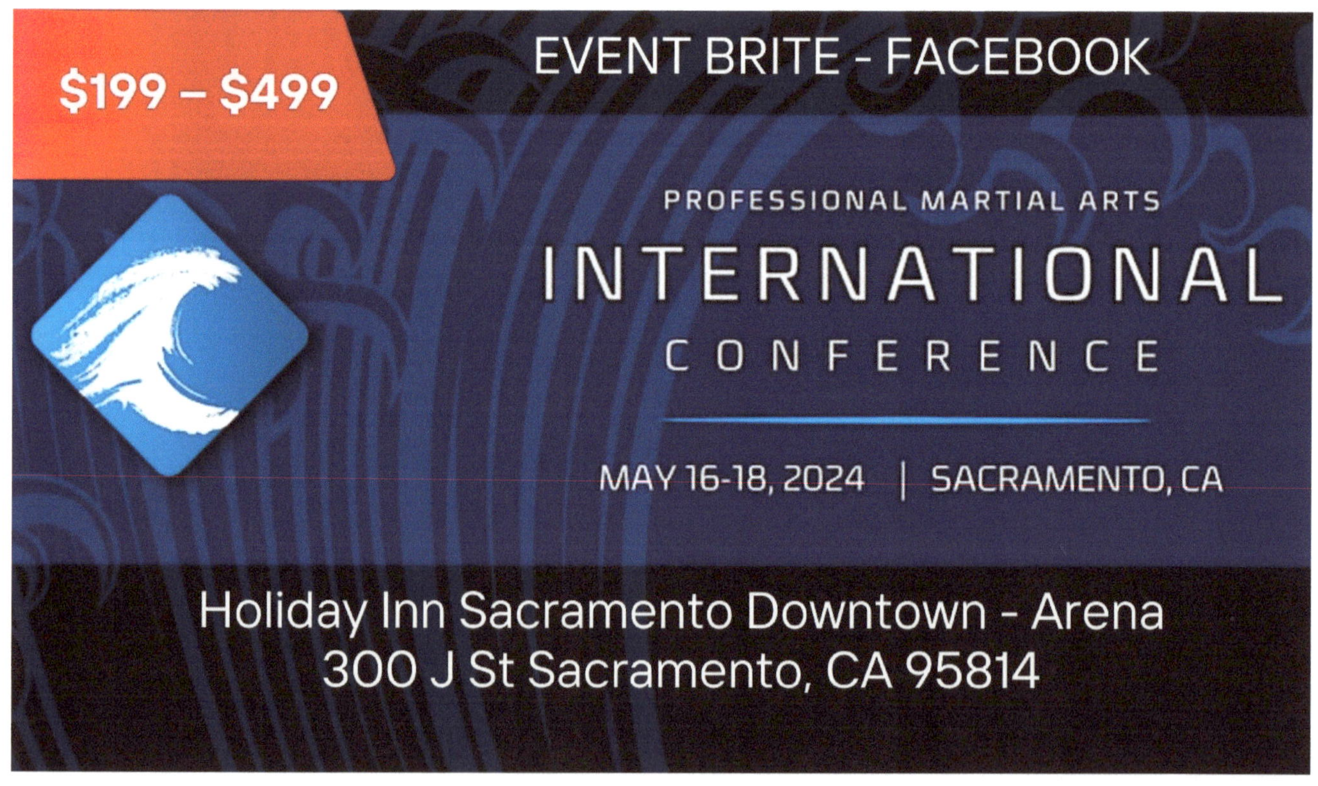

Musashi's Dokkodo
The Way of the Lone Warrior

Available on March 17!
Get Your Copy on Amazon.com
or Preorder Your Signed Copy
on TheWisdomWarrior.com!

Bohdi Sanders, Ph.D.
Author of the #1 Bestseller MODERN BUSHIDO
Foreword by Martial Arts Legend Sifu Al Dacascos

THE HEALING TOUCH

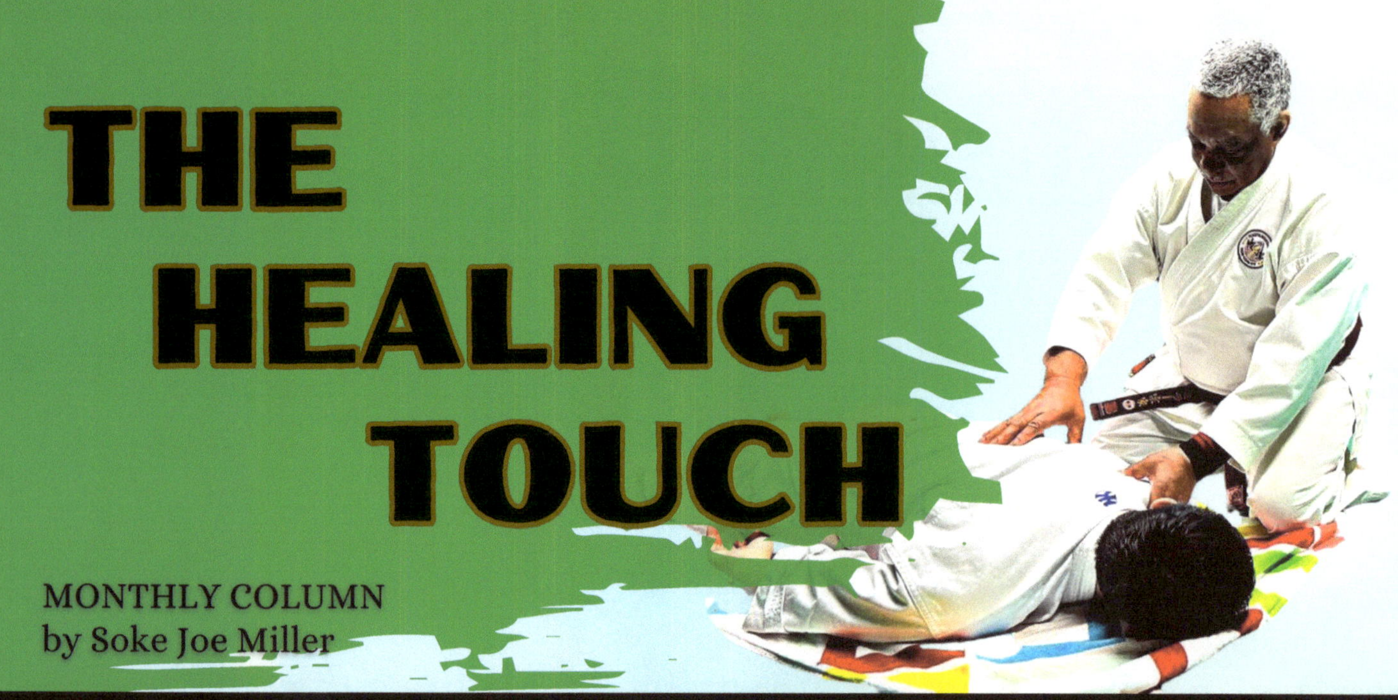

MONTHLY COLUMN
by Soke Joe Miller

THE YIN & YANG OF HEALING

The yin and yang symbol, also known as Taijitu, is deeply embedded in martial arts philosophy. In the context of health and healing, the symbol represents the balance of complementary forces. Yin and yang elements are seen in the dynamic balance of movements, the interplay of offense and defense, and the management of energy or 'Qi' in martial arts practices.

The goal is to harmonize these forces within the body to promote physical and mental well-being, and to enhance healing. To delve deeper into these concepts, martial arts practitioners often integrate meditation, controlled breathing, and Qi Gong exercises into their training, all of which are believed to foster health and recovery.

Yin and yang as it brings into healing and the martial arts.

Introduction to Shiatsu and Meridian Lines

• Shiatsu: A form of Japanese bodywork based on concepts in traditional Chinese medicine, including the flow of qi (energy) through meridians (pathways) in the body.

• Meridian Lines: Pathways through which the life-energy known as qi flows. These lines connect specific organs and are central to both healing practices and martial arts in Asian traditions. be present in all aspects of life and the universe.

• Application in Shiatsu: Shiatsu practitioners aim to balance yin and yang within the body to promote health and well-being.

Shiatsu's Approach to Health and Healing

 • Diagnosis and Treatment: Practitioners use diagnosis methods based on traditional Chinese medicine to identify imbalances in the meridian lines.

• Techniques: Application of pressure, stretches, and manipulations to specific points along the meridian lines to balance yin and yang, enhance the flow of qi, and promote health

Better Health through Harmonized Energy

• Preventive and Curative Aspects: By maintaining balance in the body's energy system, shiatsu helps in preventing illness and treating conditions ranging from stress to musculoskeletal problems.

• Holistic Approach: Emphasizes the connection between mind, body, and spirit in the pursuit of health and wellness.

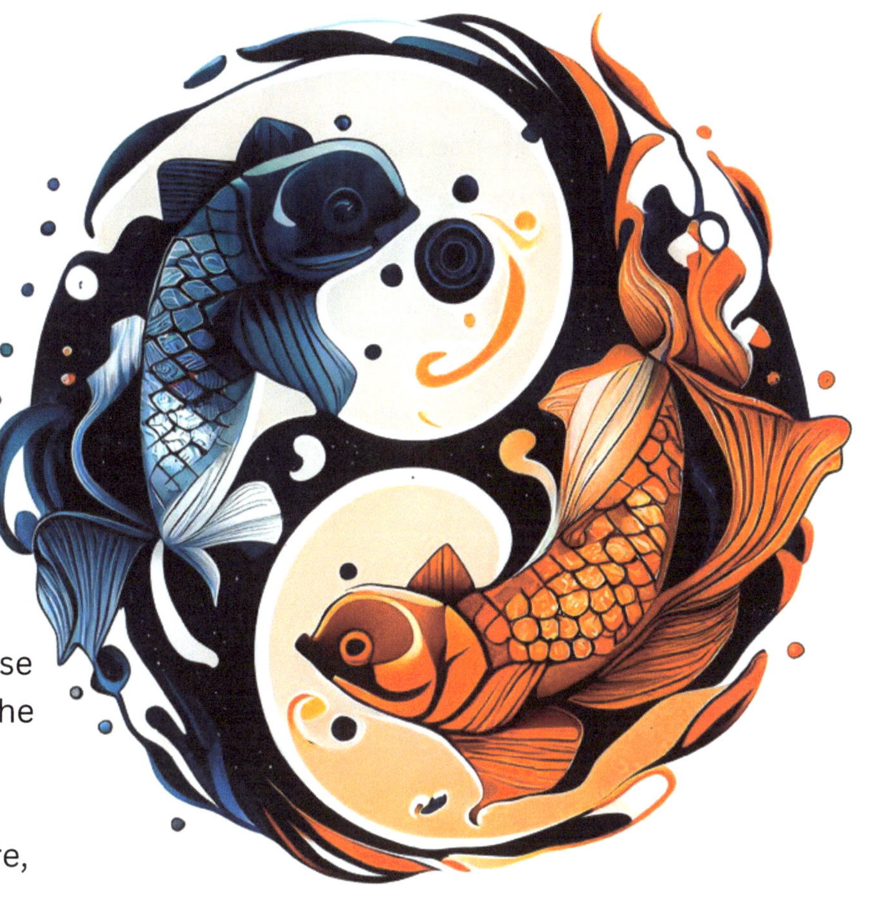

Connection between Shiatsu, Meridian Lines, and Martial Arts

• Shared Knowledge: Both shiatsu and martial arts like Aikido or Kung Fu and Jujutsu utilize an understanding of meridian lines to achieve their goals—whether for healing or for defense.

• Meridian Lines in Martial Arts: Knowledge of these lines is used to strike or manipulate specific points that can either incapacitate an opponent or, conversely, be used to heal.

Martial Arts: Defense and Healing • Dual Use of Pressure Points:

Just as pressure points can be targeted for healing in shiatsu, they can also be used in martial arts to apply strikes or holds that can disable an opponent.

• Energy Manipulation: The concept of manipulating energy (qi) for self-defense or to neutralize attacks without causing permanent damage.

Conclusion: Integrative Practices for Well-being

• Holistic Health and Self-Defense: The integrated approach of using meridian lines for both health and martial arts illustrates a deep understanding of the body's energy system.

• Lifelong Practice: Both shiatsu and martial arts offer paths toward better health, self-discipline, and understanding of the natural balance within and around us. This outline captures the essence of how shiatsu, yin and yang, and the martial arts interconnect through the concept of meridian lines, serving both as a means to foster health and as a foundation for defense techniques.

Soke Joe Miller is a highly experienced martial artist who has dedicated a significant portion of his life to studying and teaching various martial arts. He has synthesized his extensive knowledge and experience into his own system called Taizan Ryu, the Peaceful Mountain System.

This system not only focuses on self-defense techniques but also emphasizes the importance of the healing arts, such as the specific form of Shiatsu he has developed. His philosophy underscores the commitment required to maintain proficiency in martial arts, and he highlights the necessity of being able to defend oneself from any direction, recognizing that martial arts are a way of life.

He lives and runs his own Peaceful Mountain school in Hachioji, Japan with his wife Yuri.

For any questions or comments please contact him directly through facebook or social media outlets or go to his website

Contact Soke Joe Miller directly
www.peacefulmountainsystemtaizanryu.site

★★★★★ Tony B.

That's a really good book. Picture, text, Everything is so detailed

★★★★★ Kennete Kleese

The book is understandable whether you are a beginner or advance student or professional of any style of massage

★★★★★ Barry Southam

Great text to add to your library.

Learn the ancient art of shiatsu massage and its healing abilities.Relieve stress and aches while healing the body naturally through the Japanese art of acute finger pressure through this insightful and useful guide. With full-color photos and artwork of the human anatomy and step by step practice guides to instruct you from student to fully certified practitioner. In Japan, the practice of finger pressure massage known as Shiatsu is a highly respected, professional skill that uses the meridians and blood flow to naturally heal the body. Shiatsu can reduce tension and even alleviate health issues. Includes Test out portions of the text to gain full credentials in this amazing healing method from Asia.

LIMITED
$69.95
FREE DELIVERY

- Language : English
- Paperback : 299 pages
- Dimensions : 7 x 0.71 x 10 inches

QUALITY GUARANTEED

AVAILABLE ON AMAZON.COM

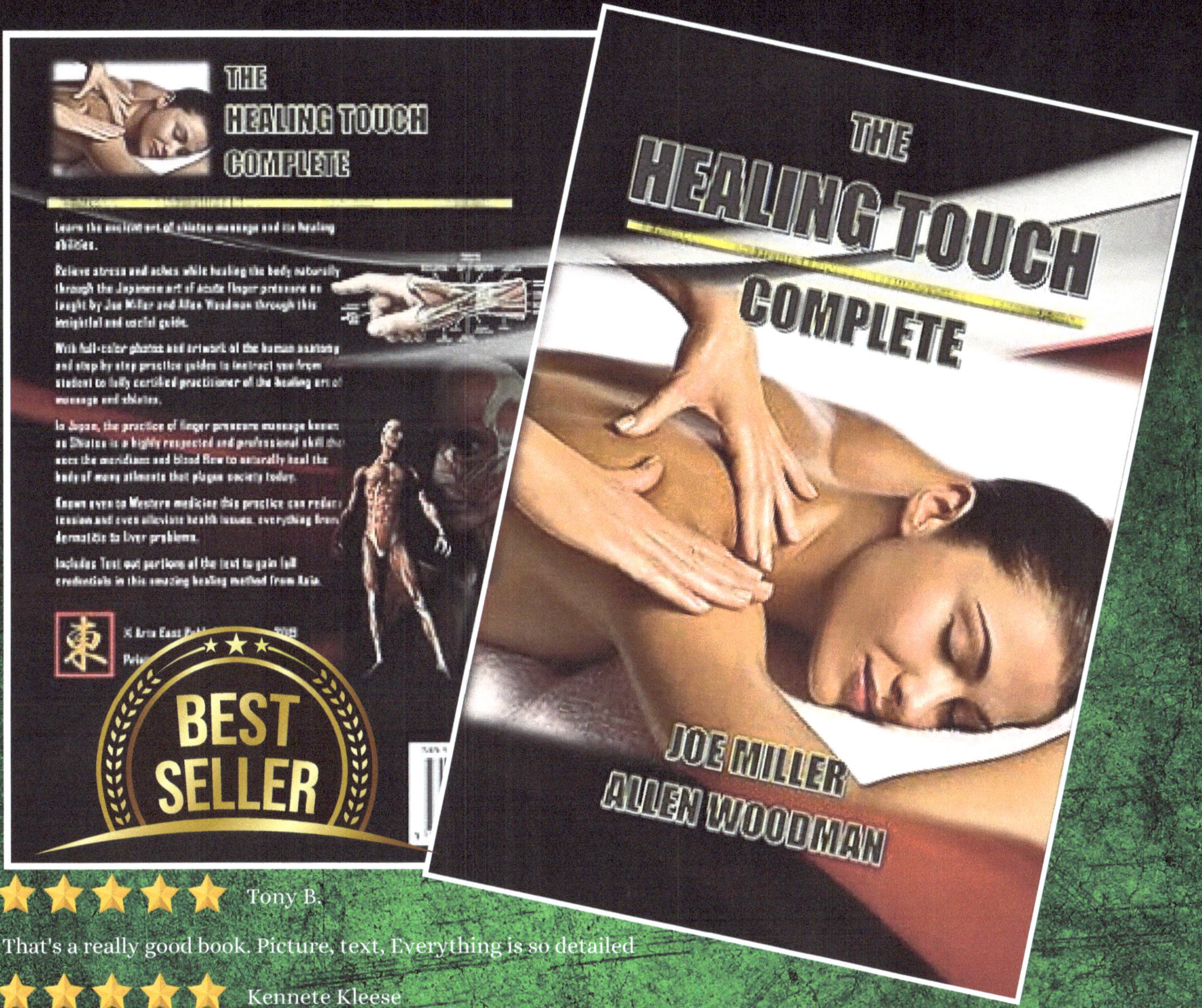

JKD
GUARDING THE GATE

WRITTEN BY
GEORGE HAJNASR
PHOTOGRAPHS BY MARY NEVINS

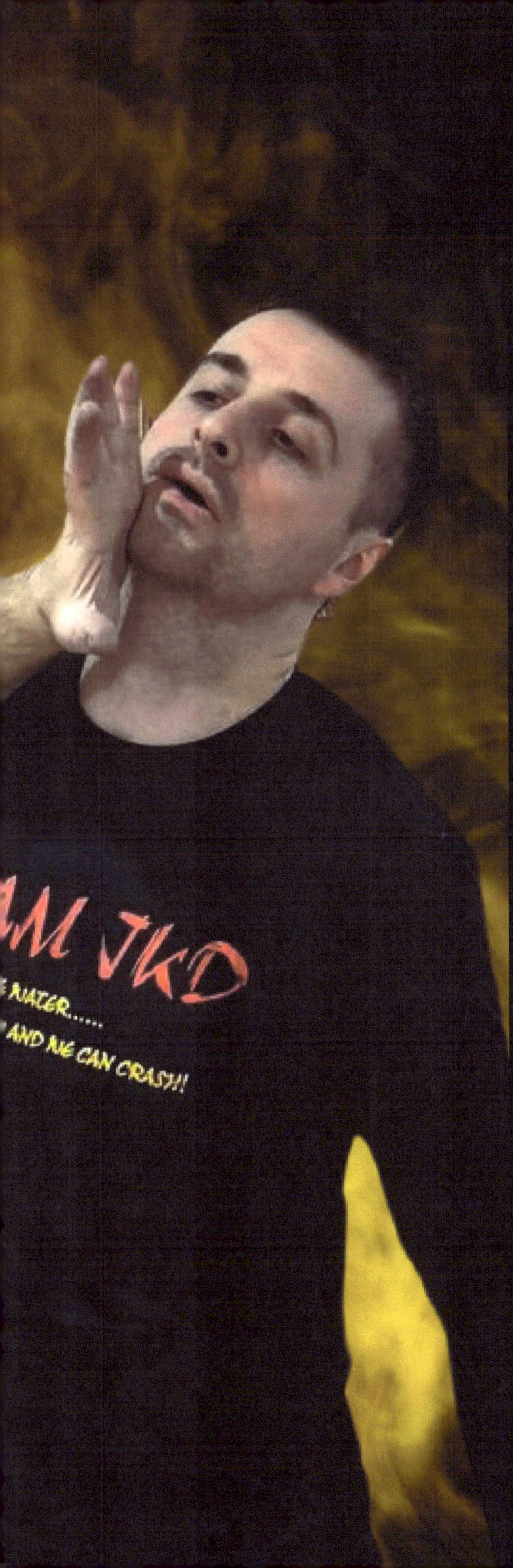

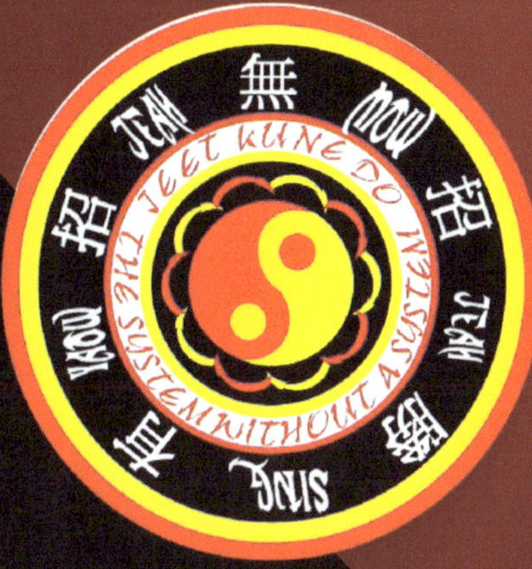

**Excerpts from
JKD System
without a system
by Geroge Hajnasr**

Born and raised in Zahle, Lebanon, George Hajnasr's passion for martial arts was ignited at a young age. After immigrating to the United States in 1981, he dedicated himself to training in Bruce Lee's teachings. Through years of hard work and education, George evolved into a skilled martial arts instructor and practitioner, specializing in the art of Jeet Kune Do. Alongside his martial arts journey, George also pursued a successful career as a master jeweler, showcasing his expertise in diamonds, precious metals, and custom creations. George's fascination with Bruce Lee's art led him to embark on a journey of martial arts training. After extensive research, he began his serious training in disciplines such as Kickboxing, Boxing, Kenpo, Shotokan, Aikido, Karate, and Jiu Jitsu. However, it was Jeet Kune Do that captured his heart, inspiring him to write and trademark his own interpretation of the art, becoming the founder of Jeet Kune Do "The System Without A System.®" George's dedication to Jeet Kune Do led him to train with renowned instructors and practitioners, including Sifu Ted Wong, Dan Inosanto, Taky Kimura, and Richard Bustillo. George's passion for Jeet Kune Do extended beyond his personal training.

Born and raised in Zahle, Lebanon, George Hajnasr's passion for martial arts was ignited at a young age. After immigrating to the United States in 1981, he dedicated himself to training in Bruce Lee's teachings. Through years of hard work and education, George evolved into a skilled martial arts instructor and practitioner, specializing in the art of Jeet Kune Do. Alongside his martial arts journey, George also pursued a successful career as a master jeweler, showcasing his expertise in diamonds, precious metals, and custom creations. George's fascination with Bruce Lee's art led him to embark on a journey of martial arts training. After extensive research, he began his serious training in disciplines such as Kickboxing, Boxing, Kenpo, Shotokan, Aikido, Karate, and Jiu Jitsu. However, it was Jeet Kune Do that captured his heart, inspiring him to write and trademark his own interpretation of the art, becoming the founder of Jeet Kune Do "The System Without A System.®" George's dedication to Jeet Kune Do led him to train with renowned instructors and practitioners, including Sifu Ted Wong, Dan Inosanto, Taky Kimura, and Richard Bustillo. George's passion for Jeet Kune Do extends far beyond his personal training.

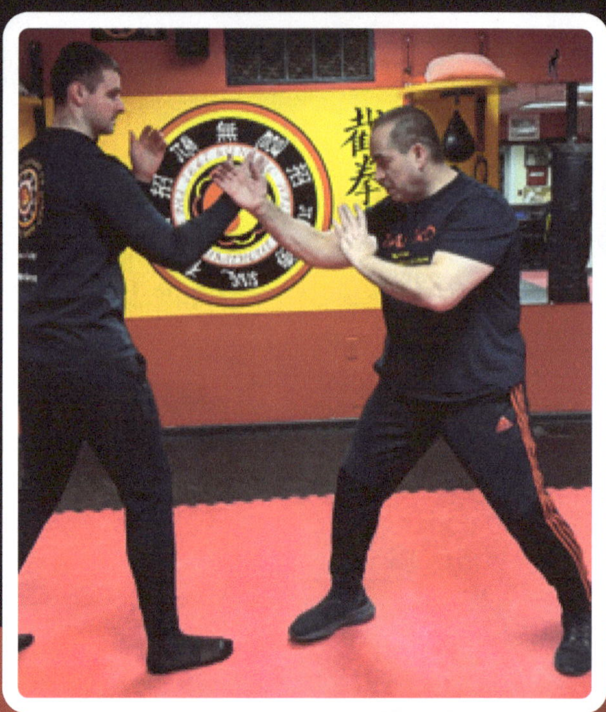

Gate (1) Both Practitioners in a Bi Jon (On Guard) Position .Woo Sau (Guarding Hand) Pock Sau Choon Choy (Push straight punch)

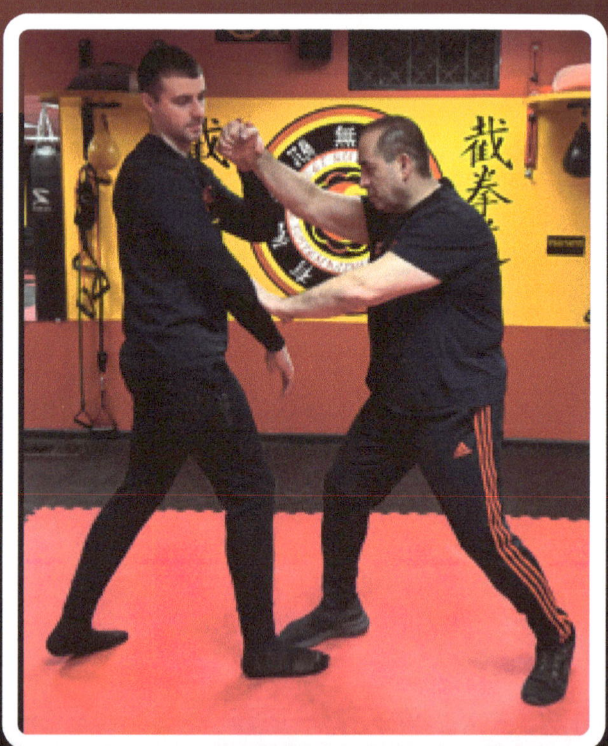

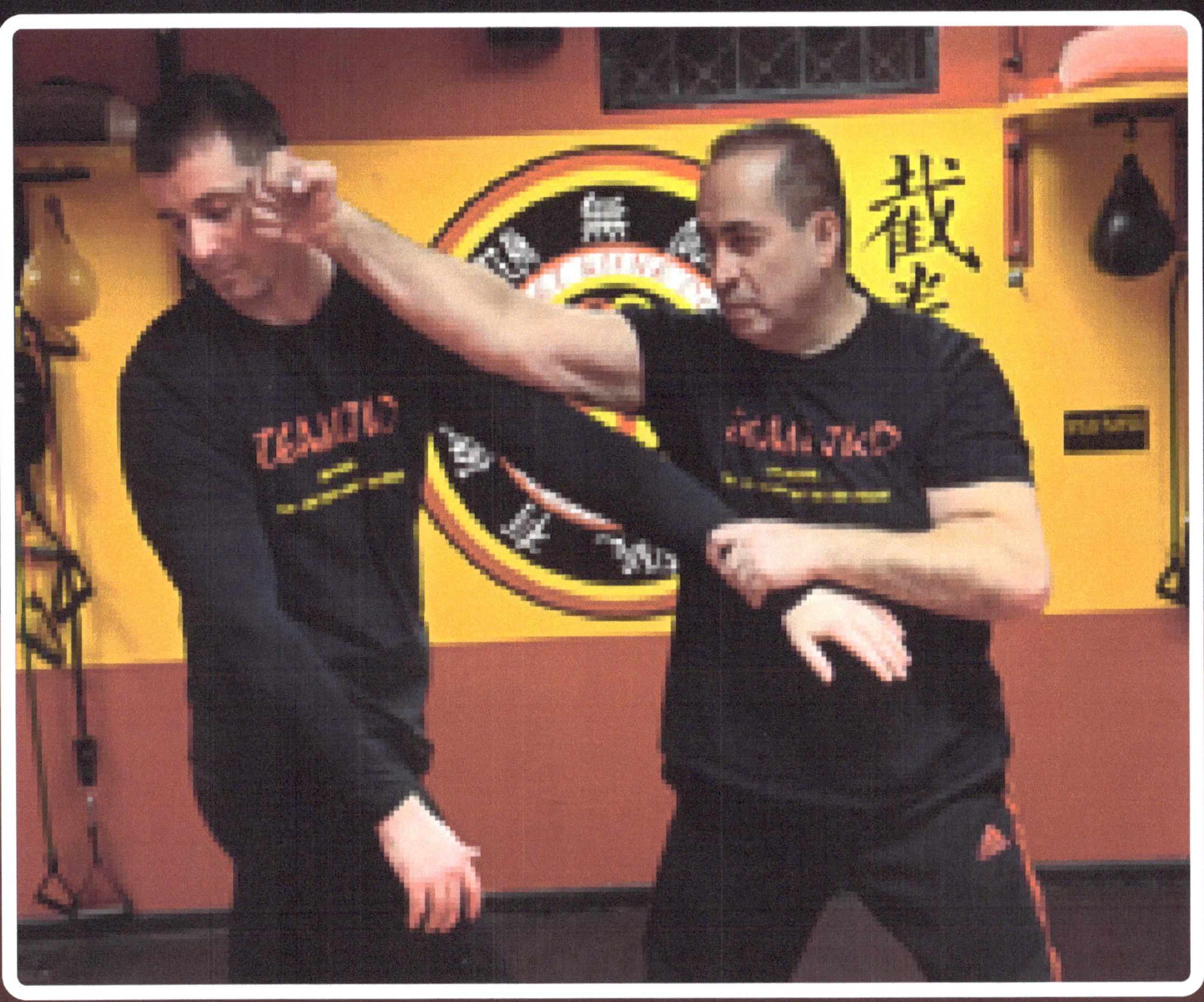

In this article, we delve into the concept of gates in Jeet Kune Do (JKD) and how they can be utilized to intercept and counter an opponent's attacks. We explore the various techniques and strategies involved in breaking down these gates and immobilizing the opponent's blocking hand. Additionally, we emphasize the importance of mastering these gates as they form the foundation of JKD training.

Understanding Gates:

Gates, also referred to as doors or openings of opportunity, are the points at which interception occurs in JKD. As the opponent strikes, we intercept either at the opening or during the retraction of their attack.

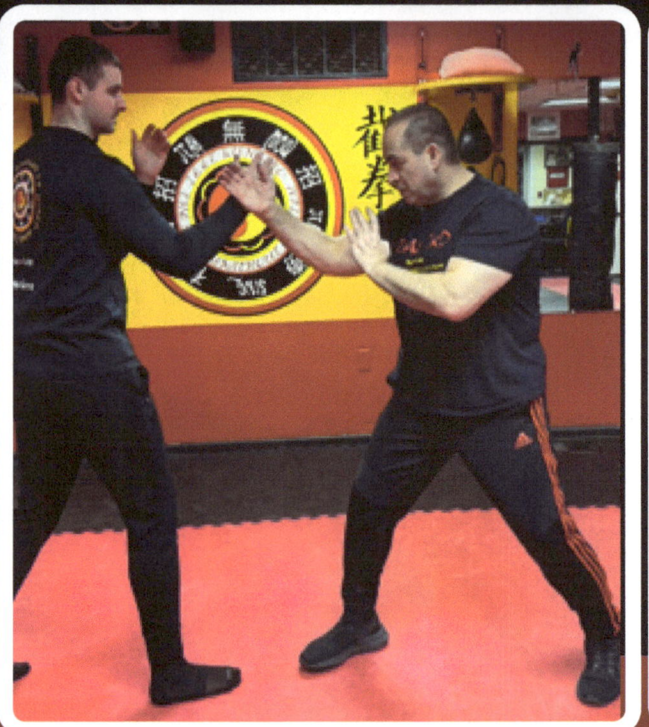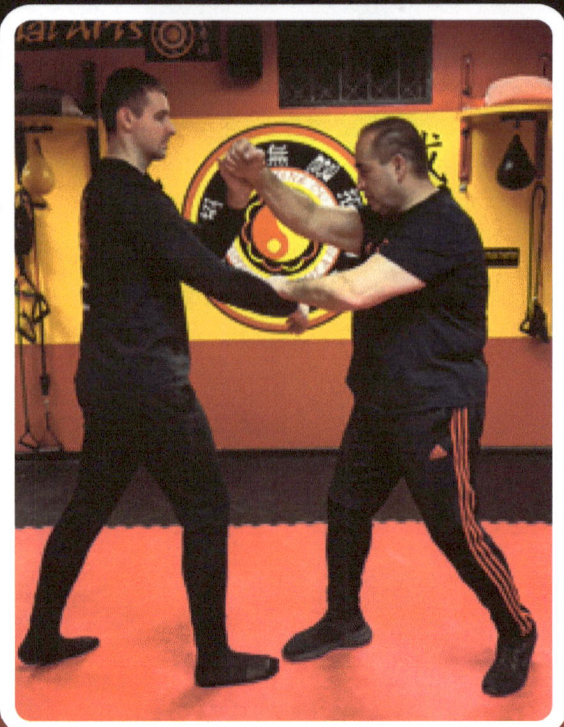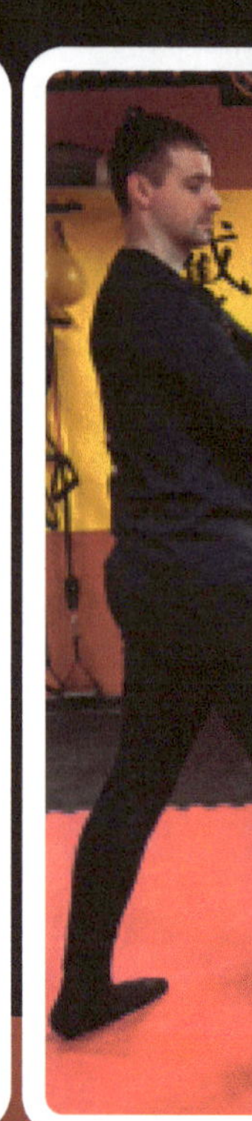

**Gate (2) Both Practitioners in a Bi Jon (On Guard) Position .
Woo Sau (Guarding Hand)**

Techniques for Breaking Down Gates:

There are several ways to break down gates in JKD, including Single Direct Attack (SDA), Hand Immobilization Attack (HIA), Trapping Hand (FON SOW), Attack By Combination (ABC), Progressively Indirect Attack (PIA), Attack By Drawing (ABD), and closing in on the attacker to neutralize their entire weapon. These techniques provide a powerful force capable of overcoming any defense, regardless of how well protected the opponent may be.

Mastering the Gates:

In this article, we demonstrate several gates, there are 27 in total, a number chosen in recognition of Bruce Lee's birthday. While these gates are crucial to JKD training, they should not limit practitioners to only these techniques. JKD offers unlimited techniques that can be customized, combined, and enhanced with kicks, takedowns, and other moves. The key is to become proficient in these techniques so that they become second nature in real-life situations.

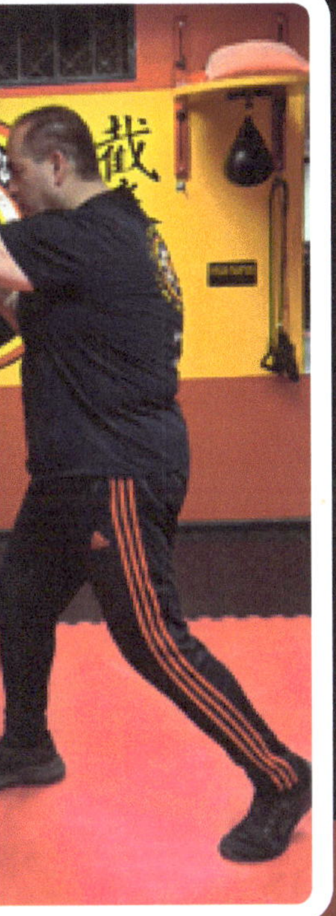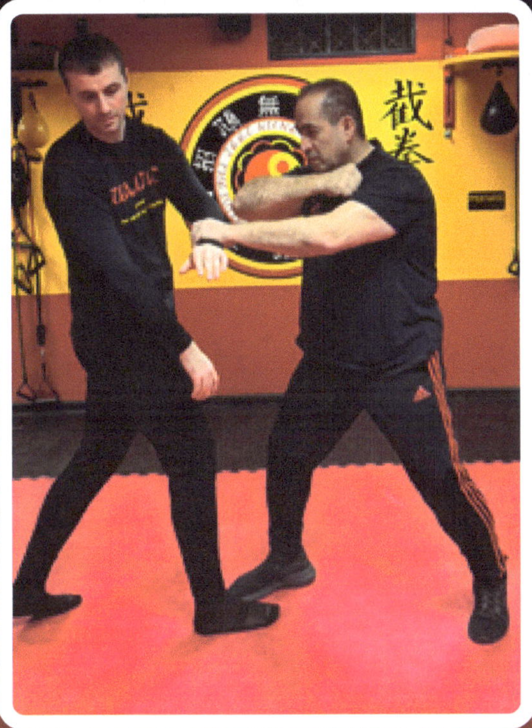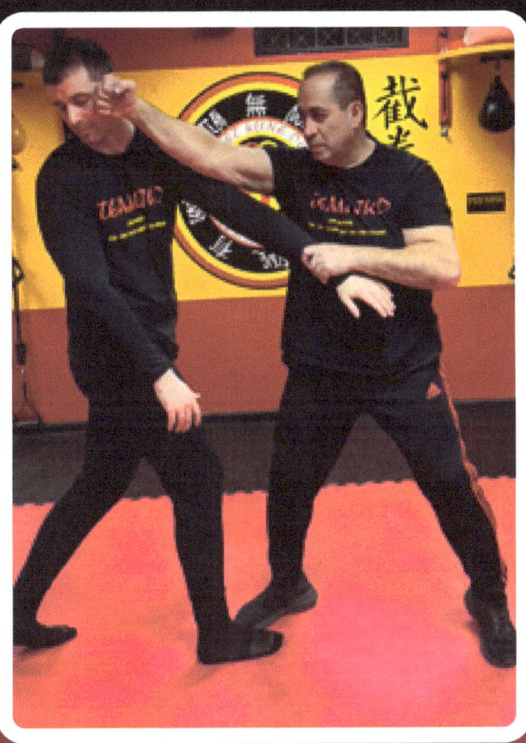

**Pock Sau Choon Choy (Push straight punch) Lop Sau (Grab Pull)
Gwa Choy (BackHand)**

Starting from Block Position:

The Importance of Footwork and Hip Rotation:

While fights don't always start from a block position, starting in this position during training allows both partners to gain valuable repetition and be one step ahead. Moreover, since 95% of people strike with their right hand, these gates are designed to counter orthodox fighters. By taking advantage of their telegraphic attacks and trapping their hands, JKD practitioners can effectively utilize the front lead position for maximum power and speed.

To achieve optimal results, footwork, pivoting, and hip rotation play a significant role in executing the gates. Practitioners must maintain a right lead unless they are left-handed. Striking from the rear can diminish power and lead to self-trapping, as it goes against the Yin and Yang structure of JKD. By positioning the right hand forward, practitioners gain power and speed, making it challenging for opponents to block even the first strike.

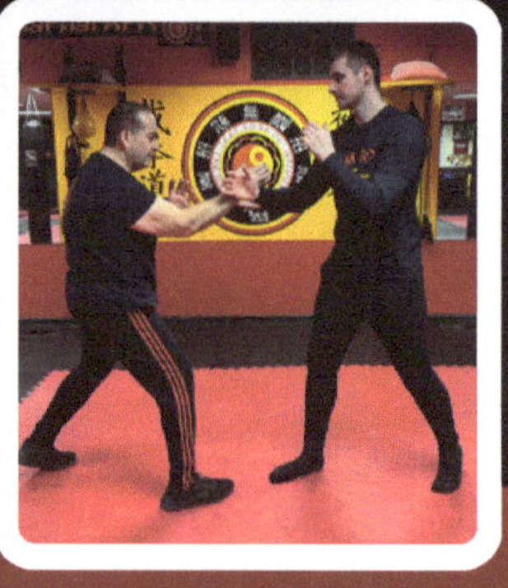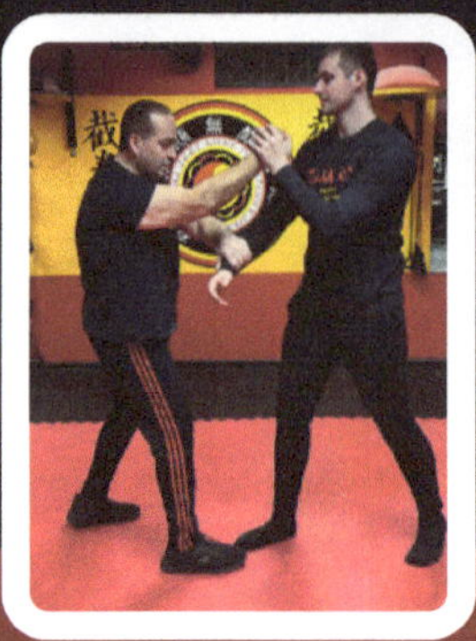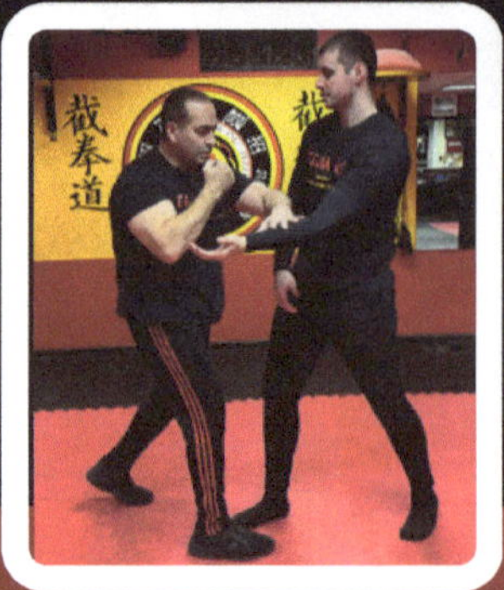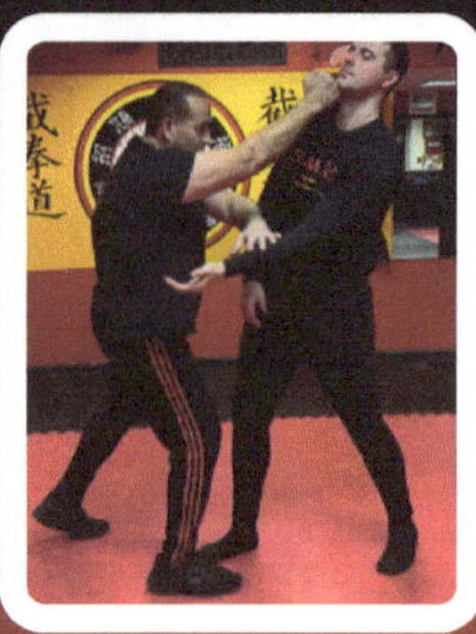

Gate (3) Both Practitioners in a Bi Jon (On Guard) Position .Woo Sau (Guarding Hand) Pock Sau choon kune (Push punch) Cow Sau Chey Kune (Catch Straight lead Punch)

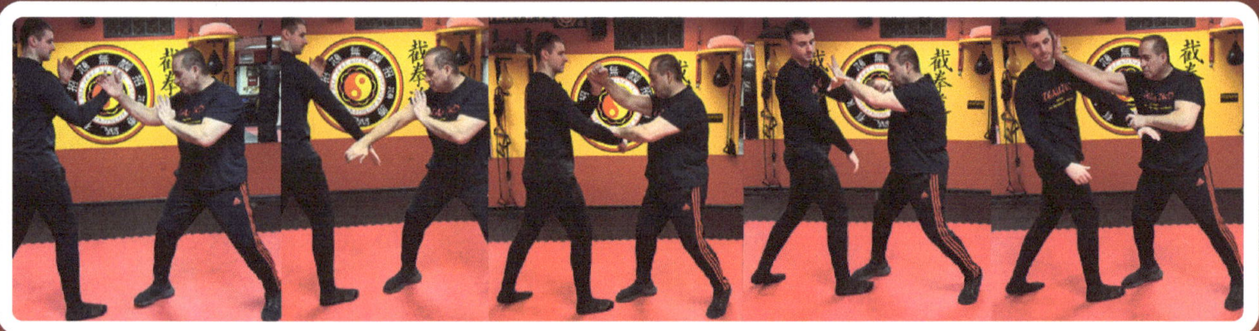

Gate (4) Both Practitioners in a Bi Jon (On Guard) Position .Woo Sau (Guarding Hand) Chop Choy (Low Strike) Gum Sau (Pin) Gwa Choy (Back Hand) Lop Sau (Grab Pull) Jow Sau (Running Hand)

Leak Attacks and Countermeasures:

A leak attack refers to an opponent's attempt to land an attack between the lower and upper defense lines, even when the gates are well closed. Skilled JKD practitioners possess the ability to find openings and execute these attacks with speed, snap, and precise footwork. By practicing the gates, JKD punches become "felt before they are seen," enhancing the practitioner's overall effectiveness.

Mastering the gates in JKD is essential for intercepting and countering an opponent's attacks. By understanding the various techniques and strategies involved, practitioners can break down gates, immobilize the opponent's blocking hand, and unleash powerful strikes. However, it is crucial to remember that the gates are not the only techniques available in JKD. Practitioners should adapt and combine techniques based on the situation, ultimately becoming proficient in responding naturally to any attack.

JEET KUNE DO

THE SYSTEM WITHOUT A SYSTEM

BOOK + DVD

ORDER NOW

AVAILABLE NOW

$29.95

BEST PRICE

502 pages
Language English
Publication February 3, 2014
Dimensions 8.5 x 1.01 x 11.02

Jeet Kune Do A System Without a System is one of the best books ever written on the complete system that was pioneered by the late great Bruce Lee. George Hajnasr has put together the full course and understanding principles that are the make up of the complete system. Everything from Warm Up exercises to self defense techniques ranging from beginner to advanced. You will find it all in this one large manual of the Complete system of Jeet Kune DO A System Without a System.

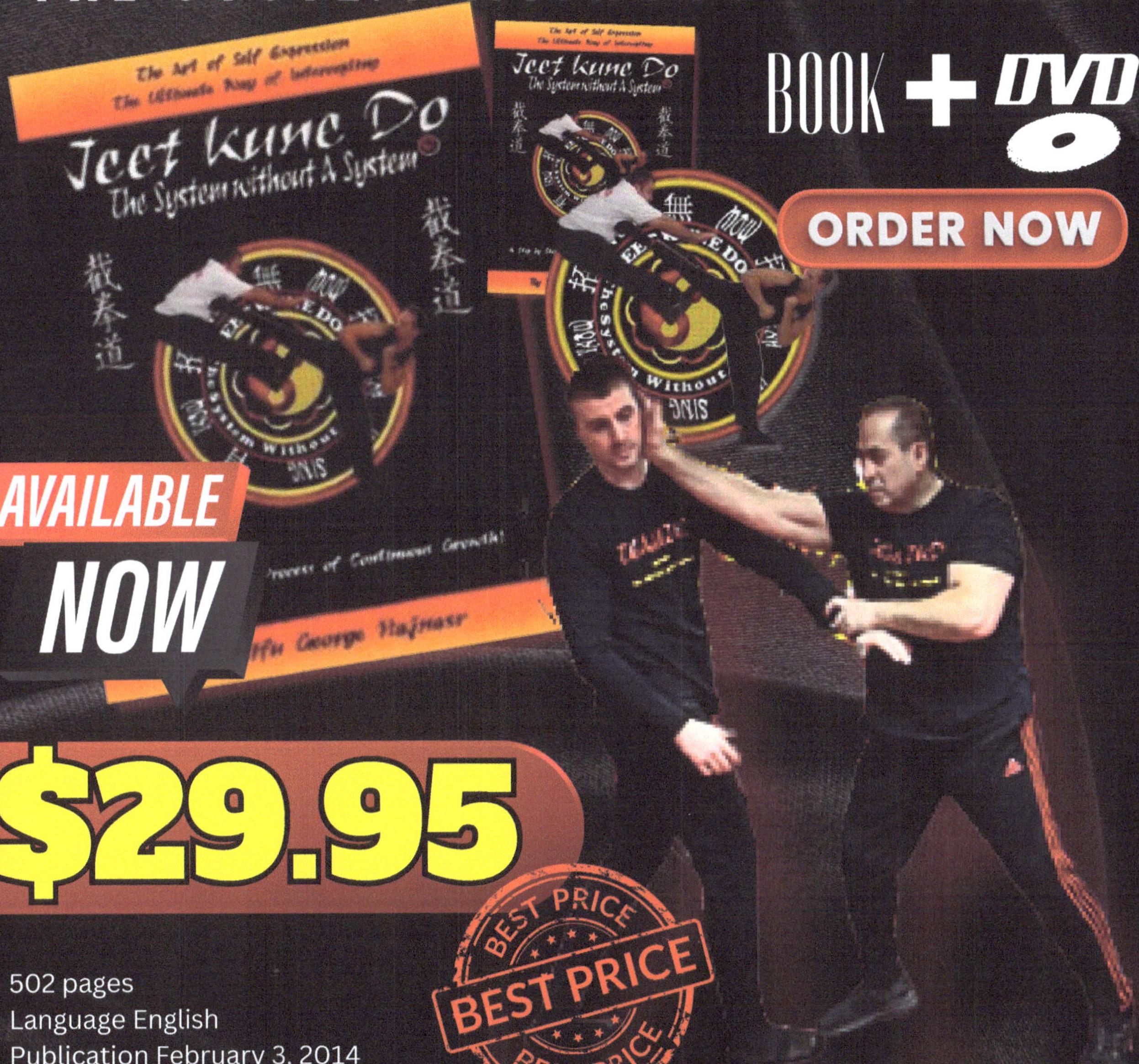

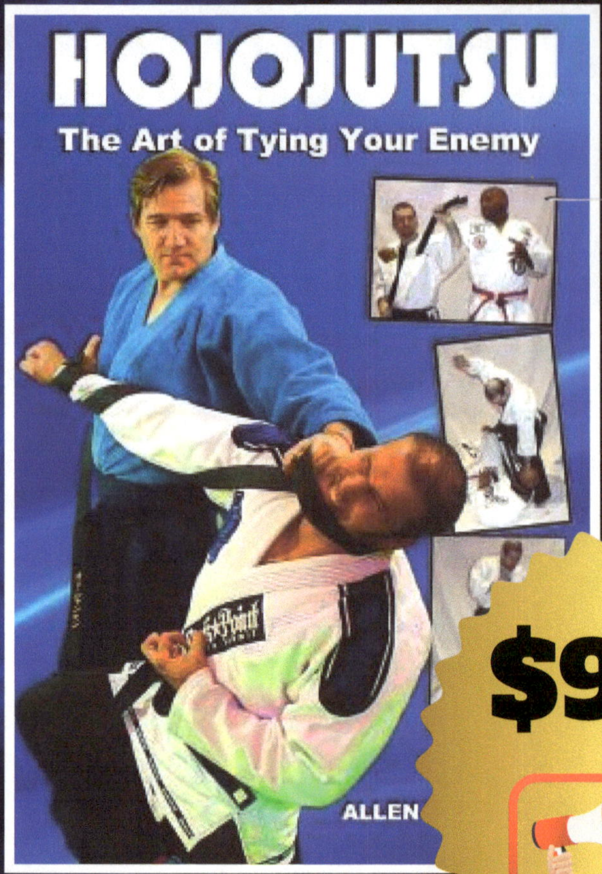

HOJOJUTSU
The Art of Tying Your Enemy

ALLEN

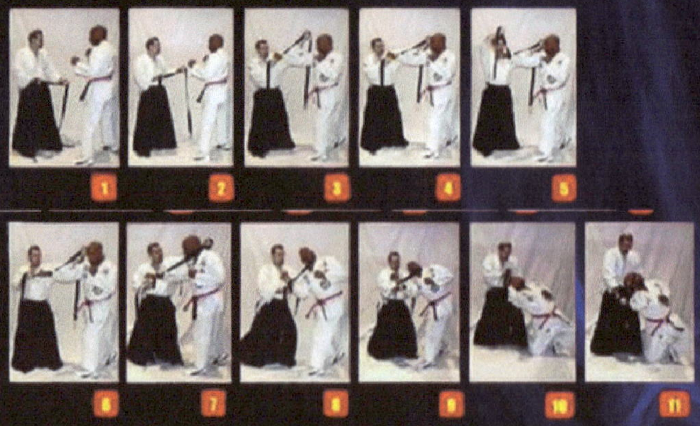

Step-By-Step Instruction

$9.95
+ S & H

TODAY ONLY

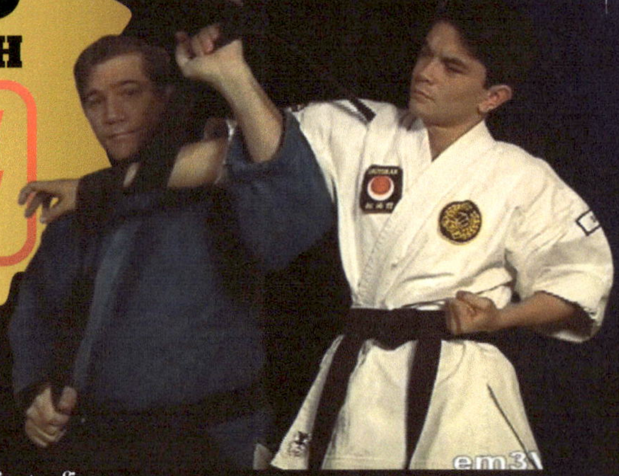

★★★★★ John Atkinson

New concept, for America, really effective

★★★★★ Richard Hopkins

The first practical account I have seen of these techniques for over forty five years.

Hojojutsu is the traditional Japanese martial art of restraining a person using cord or rope. Encompassing many different materials, techniques and methods from many different schools, Hojojutsu is quintessentially a Japanese art that is a unique product of Japanese history and culture. It is the beautiful and peculiar art of restraining someone using (often brightly colored) cord. It is rarely practiced outside of Japan and is an ancient strand of martial art with a rich and complex history. As a martial arts practice, Hojojutsu is seldom, if ever, taught on its own but as part of a curriculum under the aegis of the body of study encompassed by a larger school of bugei or budo, often as an advanced study in jujutsu. Hojojutsu techniques and methods are seldom demonstrated outside of Japan. Shihan Allen Woodman has trained over 20 years in Japan and is the Chief Instructor at the Dento Teki Na Dojo, the Kokusai Karate Do Renmei Hombu Dojo in Bronx, New York. Sensei Allen Woodman offers this book on the traditional martial art of Hojojutsu. This is one of the only books ever published on this art form detailing the defensive practices and techniques of the art.

125 pages
Language
English
Publication date
March 15, 2013
Dimensions
6.9 x 0.5 x 9.9

AVAILABLE ON AMAZON.COM

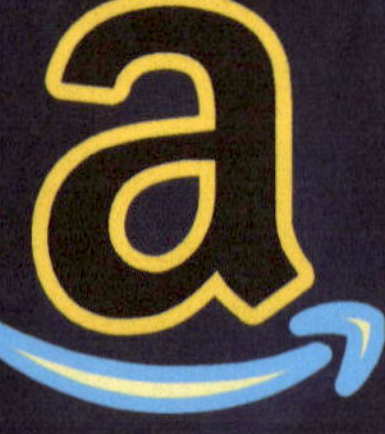

Florida Sport Taekwondo Federation State Championship

2024

USATKD Florida State Championships

April 27th, 2024

Sarasota Fairgrounds

3000 Ringling Blvd
Sarasota, Fl 34237

Florida Sport Taekwondo Federation
Chairman and CEO Master Mark Antonucci, Director Master Dennis White,
Director Master Russell Beneby, Director Master James White, Director Master Angelito Ong,
Referee Chairman Master Jin Hwan Hwang

To Register go to
https://usataekwondo.sport80.com/public/wizard/e/288

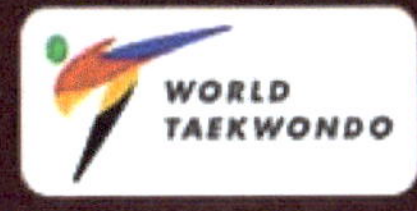

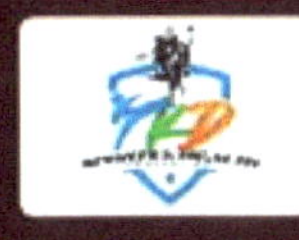

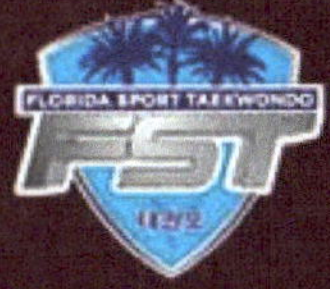

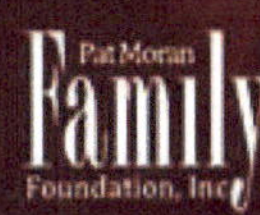

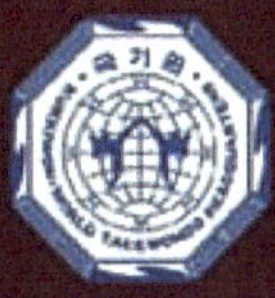

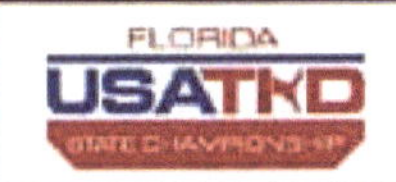

Scan QR code
for
Registration

Contact Us: 561-231-9294 / Info@FLaTKD.com   More Info www.FlaTKD.com

FRANK DUX

The Legend of BLOODSPORT

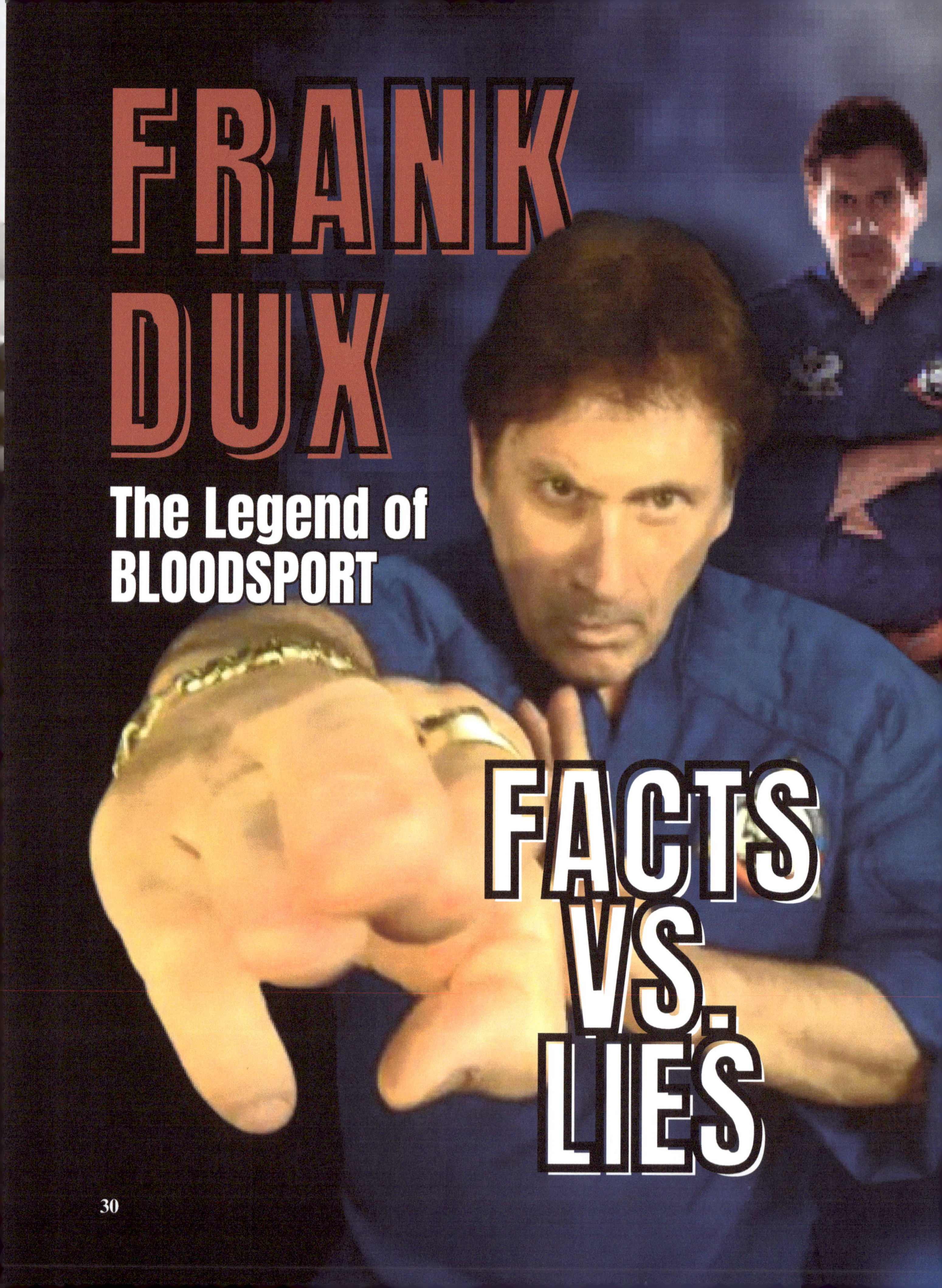

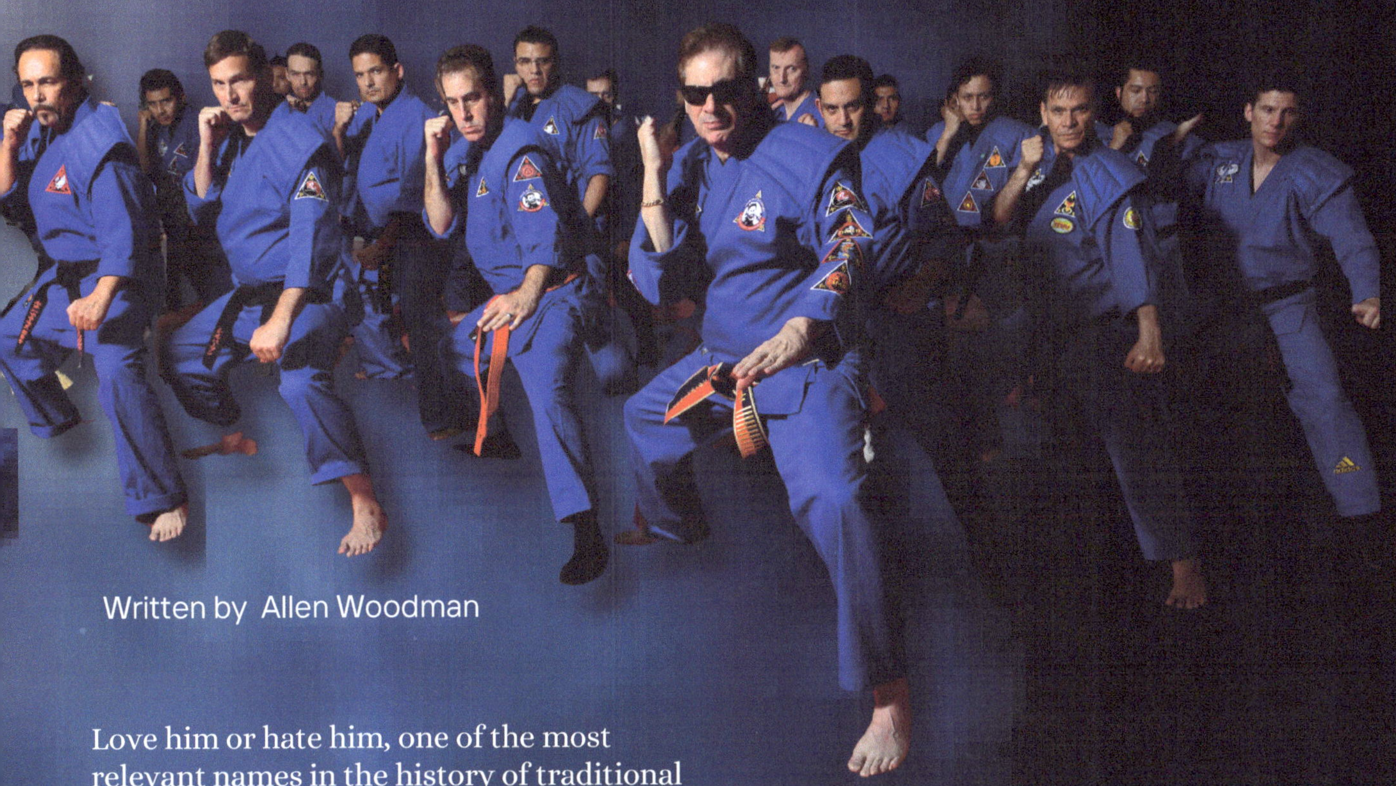

Written by Allen Woodman

Love him or hate him, one of the most relevant names in the history of traditional Asian and modern era martial arts is Bloodsport's, Frank W. Dux.

At first glance the meme: "FACEBOOK TOOK DOWN A CHUCK NORRIS POST SO CHUCK NORRIS TOOK DOWN FACEBOOK. THEN FRANK DUX MADE CHUCK PUT IT BACK UP,". It seems all in good fun.

In the world of martial arts, there are two distinct realms: the intense and violent military world, and the more ethereal and entertaining world. Frank Dux is a name that is considered iconic in both of these realms.

This duality is why he has the most impactful name in martial arts history.

In the bustling nexus where facts versus fantasy collide with the fighting spirit, a name echoes through the halls of martial arts history—Frank William Dux.

Like a whispered legend, Dux's legacy entwines the traditional art forms of ancient Asia with the dazzling neon glow of modern action cinema.

Frank Dux stands as a polarizing figure, a catalyst in the evolution of combat sports.

Enter the arena of Bloodsport, the 1988 cult classic that catapulted the notion of mixed martial arts into the global consciousness. At its heart, the enigmatic Frank Dux both inspired the story and orchestrated its ballet of violence. Against the backdrop of a skeptical Hollywood, skeptical that action films had run their course, Bloodsport soared, defying all odds with a gripping narrative and kinetic choreography courtesy of Dux himself.

With a shoestring budget that would barely cover a Hollywood starlet's wardrobe, Bloodsport raked in a king's ransom, turning a tidy $1.5 million investment into a staggering $100 million, a box office and syndication triumph.

Its secret? Authenticity and fight sequences were so compelling they left audiences spellbound.

Frank Dux didn't just train Jean-Claude Van Damme; he transformed him into an icon of strength and skill. Region by region, Bloodsport seized the number one spot, reinvigorating a genre on the brink of extinction.

And yet, not all is clear in the legacy of Frank Dux. Shadows of doubt loom large as heated debates of fraudulence and claims of literary theft bubble to the surface stemming from the trade libeling of him by his corporate rivals, unable to compete with his accomplishments or claim them for themselves.

Among the voices is one of Bloodsport's three WGA-credited screenwriters, Sheldon Lettich, who contends the verbiage "Story By Sheldon Lettich." appearing in the end credit roll for Bloodsport proves this is his brainchild when to the contrary, the Written Agreement memorializes Bloodsport is NOT a creative work by Sheldon Lettich.

The reason Sheldon Lettich has his Bloodsport "Story By" credit is he negotiated this away from Frank Dux, having brought the funding source producer Mark DiSalle to his then-screenwriting partner Dux, first to take Bloodsport story to a concrete form; work titled Return of the Ninja. He registered before having ever met Lettich.

This truth is reflected in how, in place of what would have been the customary story option/purchase agreement one enters into selling a script, Sheldon Lettich entered into a Writing Services Agreement with DiSalle, where Lettich acknowledges the producers BOUGHT THE STORY (from Dux) and that Lettich was really a -- "Work For Hire." The fact that the Frank Dux Agreement is a purchase option Agreement that memorializes he retains all literary rights in which Sheldon has no equity proves outright that Bloodsport is the brainchild of Frank Dux.

More significantly, all the written agreements establish that Bloodsport could not be made fiction. Doing so resulted in a breach of contract litigation. Frank Dux vs. FM Entertainment. Canon Films and Mark DiSalle, who transferred their ownership interests to FM, did not own fictionalization rights. Furthermore, this is reflected in addendums made to Frank Dux Bloodsport Agreement that were necessary to allow for the fictionalization of certain parts in the film (i.e., Dux going AWOL to fight to honor his master).

In defaming Frank Dux, Sheldon Lettich and others claim that Frank Dux's Kumite claims have no basis in fact that he bought his trophy; there exists no proof to be found regarding his teacher Senzo Tanaka, The Black Dragons, and his Titles World Records. This doesn't exist.

In stark contrast, YouTube footage shows Frank Dux being presented by government sport regulating authorities his world titles and records in front of thousands: a free ancestory.com search proves Senzo Tanaka's existence.

Likewise, The Black Dragon Society, Kumite fighting events are equally well documented in history books and criminal prosecutions.

Overlooking how his failure to provide a based on actual event screenplay put Sheldon Lettich in breach of his Bloodsport agreement, and no breach was filed. In addition, Lettich registered his screenplay with the WGA as "Based on A True Story." A contradictory statement of fact made by him.

Taking credit for Frank Dux's intellectual property contributions didn't stop with Bloodsport for Lettich with the WGA intervening and awarding, in 1998, Frank Dux deserved "Story By" credit for Universal Studio film, "The Quest".

Lettich name on the shooting script is credited as having provided the material for it when it was Frank Dux, and this was his story.

With regard to the genesis of Bloodsport, Dux penned his original Bloodsport script in 1980, five years before Lettich's involvement. Dux registered it with Writers Guild America West under the then working title Return of The Ninja.

The Bloodsport title is the result of Canon films selling at the AFM in 1981, Enter the Ninja, and its original producers requesting the name change to avoid confusion or legal entanglements.

Further contradicting Sheldon Lettich, more hard evidence and corroborations abound, underscoring the veracity of Dux's story -- articles, a documentary, legal testimonies, and irrefutable courtroom witnesses, like former Warner Bros. VP of Marketing and Publicity Joe Sinda.
.

In various on-camera interviews, the former Warner Bros. executive describes Frank Dux hang time as having rivaled Michael Jordan. That Sinda, amongst others like Big Jim McCune, David German, and more, was on hand to witness Dux win the Kumite depicted by Bloodsport and verified by the leading martial art magazine staff in November 1980, Black Belt magazine. Sinda, having borne firsthand account of Dux's Kumite triumphs, paved the way for Warner Bros Distribution of Bloodsport.

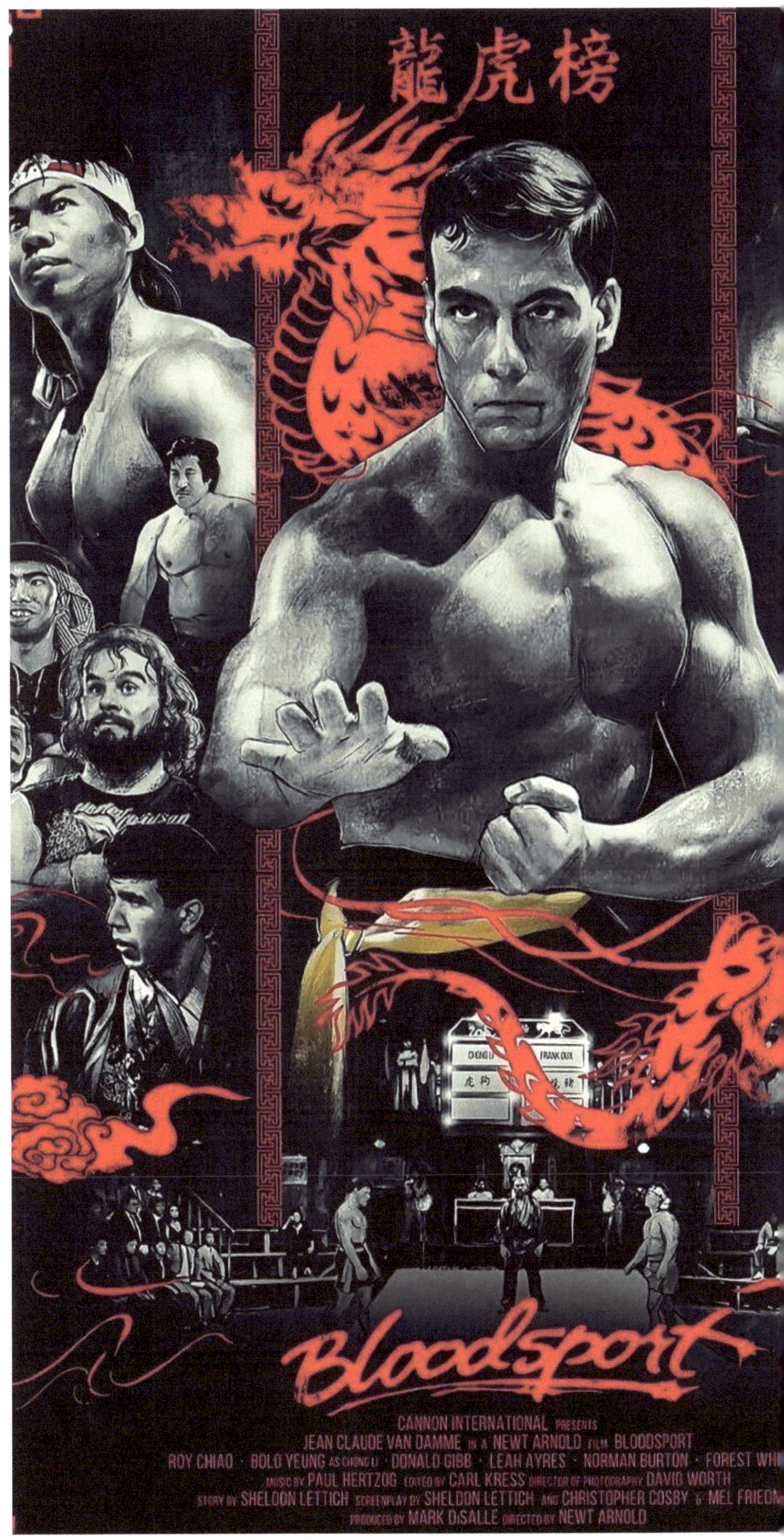

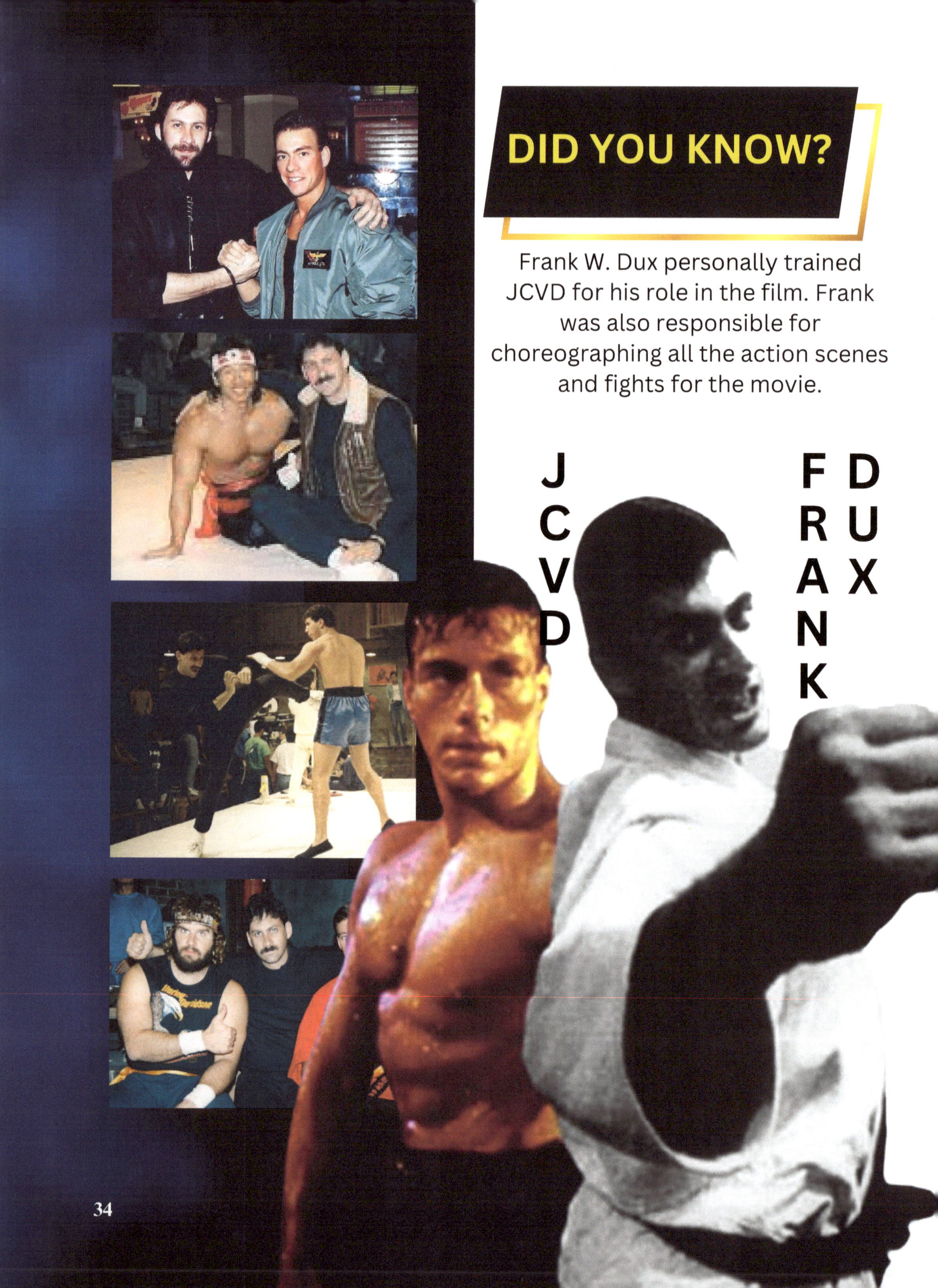

DID YOU KNOW?
Frank W. Dux personally trained JCVD for his role in the film. Frank was also responsible for choreographing all the action scenes and fights for the movie.
J
C
V
D
F
R
A
N
K
D
U
X
34

The movie "Bloodsport" which launched Jean Claude Van Dams movie career was based on the real life events of Frank W. Dux

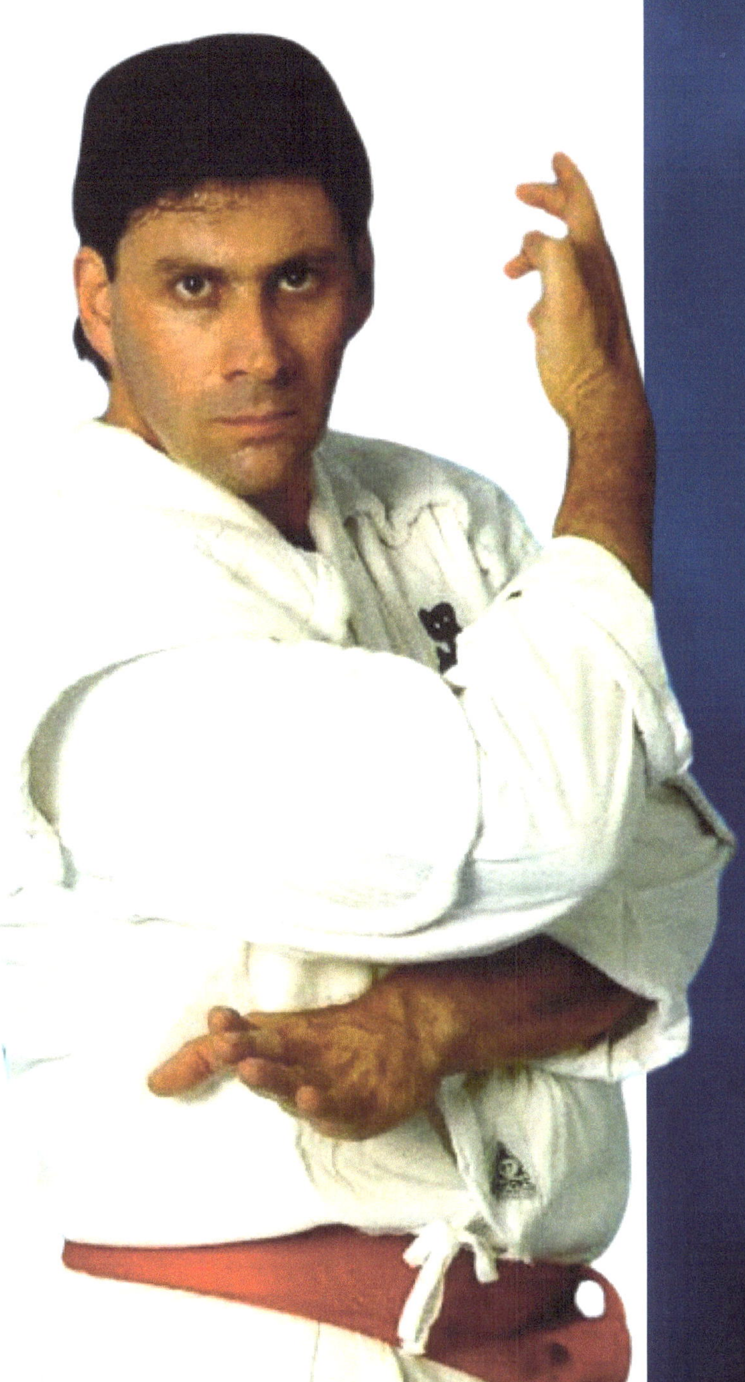

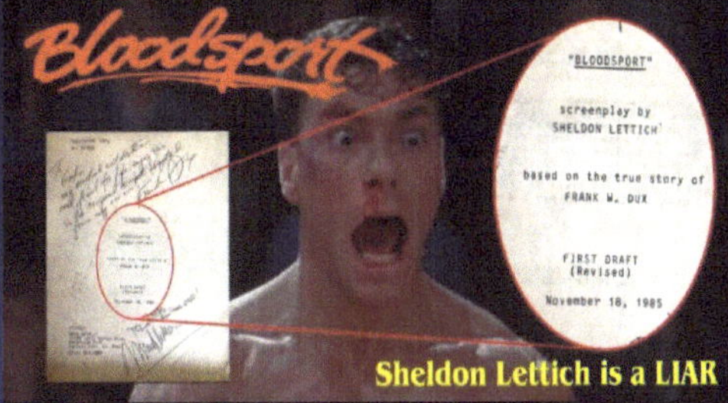

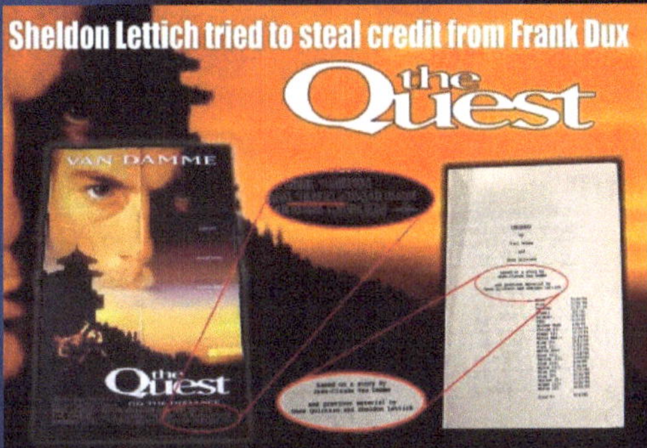

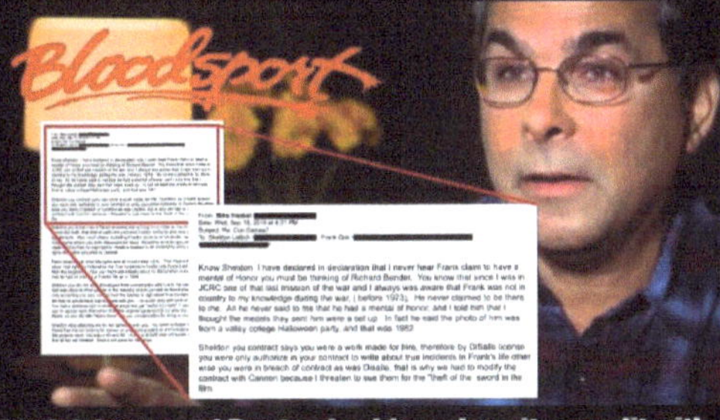

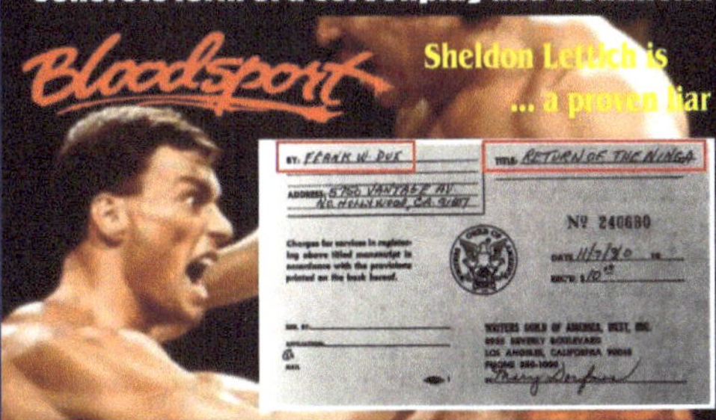

With millions for Canon Films as well as professional reputations at stake, a person must suspend logic, industry custom, and practice of performance of legal, due diligence to accept "Everyone just took Dux word for it," professed by Lettich and martial art luminaries. That benefit in creating the illusion Bloodsport is a creative work in their pigeonholing of Frank Dux. His not succumbing to this foul play is further testimony to his legend.

As unbelievable as it may seem, Dux's script satisfied the stringent criteria and critical eye of legal due diligence for truth in advertising, aligning perfectly with the movie's marketing narrative. Beyond the silver screen, Dux's influence permeates the very fabric of mixed martial arts. But to credit him solely for the creation of MMA would be to overlook the rich tapestry of fighting disciplines that the sport encompasses.

Nevertheless, Dux's contributions to popularizing martial arts cannot be overstated—with Bloodsport as the catalyst, a combat revolution was televised. In the wake of this cinematic giant, numerous films followed suit, drawing from the blueprint of Bloodsport to capture the imagination of future warriors. But beyond the lights and cameras, Frank Dux's odyssey extended to the settings of world records and martial arts festivities, sometimes facing off against the very fighters he sought to recruit for his own fighting league. This is the saga of Frank Dux—a man shrouded in myth, enshrined in celluloid, and forever ingrained in the annals of martial arts history.

As we turn the page on this chapter, one cannot help but ponder will the real Frank Dux, please stand up. Or perhaps, in the dance of light and shadow, the intrigue is the essence of his enduring allure.

DID YOU KNOW?

Dux set world records at a packed Bercy Sports Stadium in Paris France. Breaking two champaign bottles with a single kick and a palm strike through tested Bullet-proof Glass.

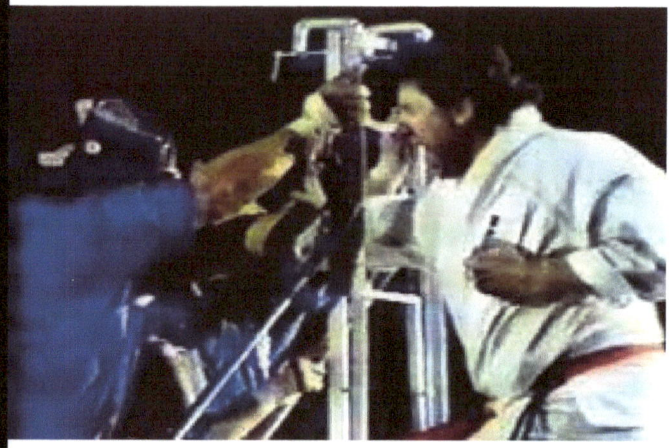

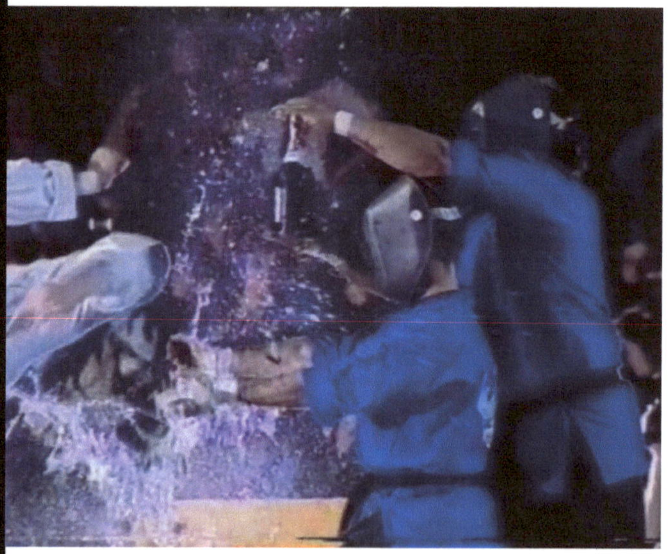

Frank Dux is listed as a contributing source in creating the U.S. Navy SEAL Special Warfare Combat Fighting course Manual

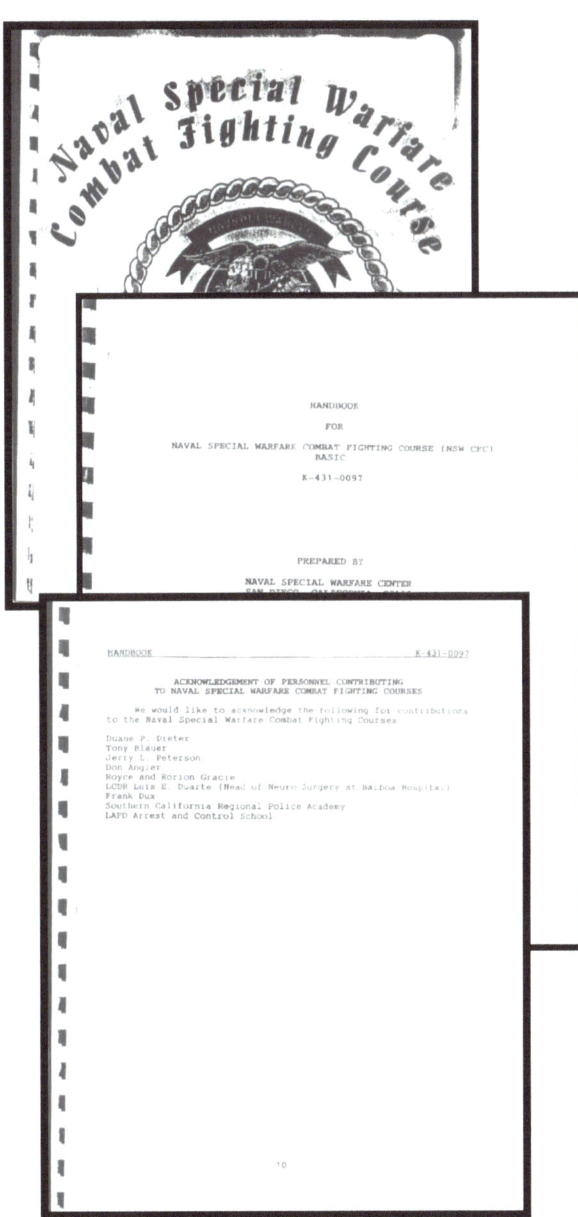

Dux's odyssey, chronicled in the pounding beats and shattered glass of "Bloodsport," transcends the glitzy veneer of Tinseltown. This martial arts maestro didn't just break box office records; he shattered real-world ones—raising the stakes, the spectacle, and the spirits of martial artists everywhere.

As we recount the adrenaline-packed exploits that saw Dux crack champagne bottles with the finesse of a seasoned sommelier and power through bullet-proof glass with his bare hands, we're not just revisiting record-breaking moments. We're diving into an era defined by a man whose life story could rival the most spellbinding of scripts.

Far from the heights of a Hollywood legend, Frank has been actively training in martial arts, opening several martial arts schools as well as training elite tactical teams. Frank Dux has been the keynote speaker for FLEOA (Federal Law Enforsment Officers association) an unprescidented 2X.

Frank W. Dux is listed as a contributing source in the Special forces SEAL team Spec Warfare Manual and has actively trained several law enforcemnt entities throughout his career.

Frank Dux didn't just usher in a new dawn for martial arts—he escorted it into the limelight with the poise of a heavyweight champion, leaving an indelible mark on the world of martial arts.

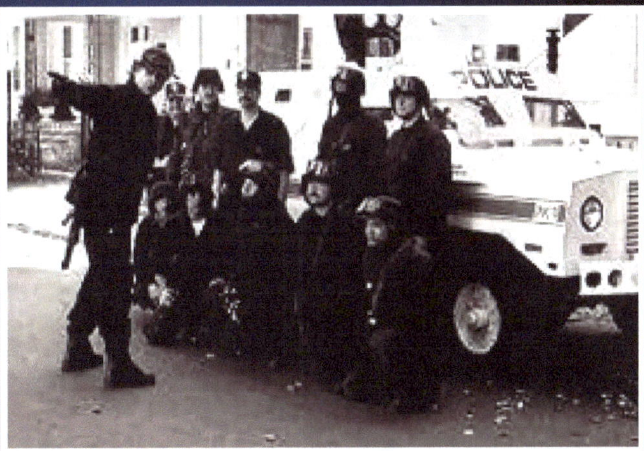

DID YOU KNOW?

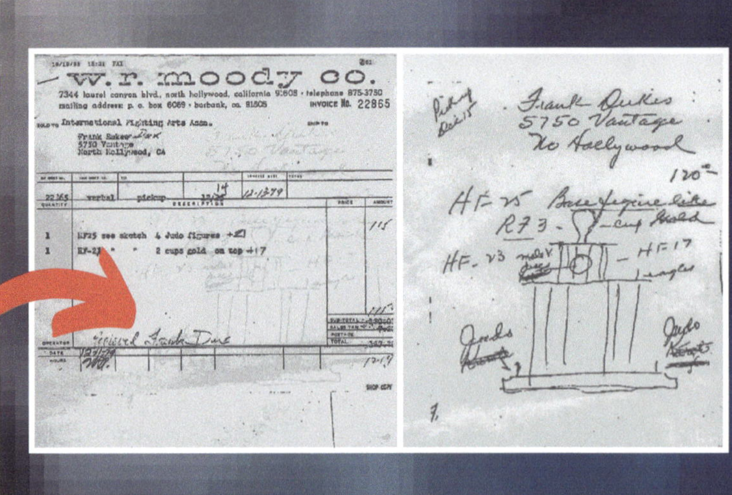

Frank Dux holds his trophy as from the infamous "Kumite"
In an attempt to debunk him, an editorial appeared with a hand drawn receipt in the L.A. Times stating that Frank bought his trophy.
Notice that the bogus receipt has the name misspelled poorly, and the hand-drawn diagram does not even resemble the trophy won.
The original photo of Frank Dux was published in Black Belt Magazine, 8 years prior to the receipt and long before the editorial was ever published.

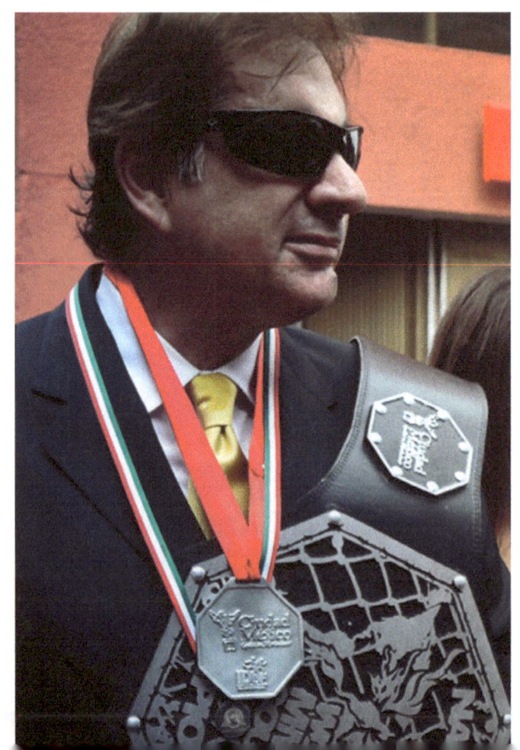

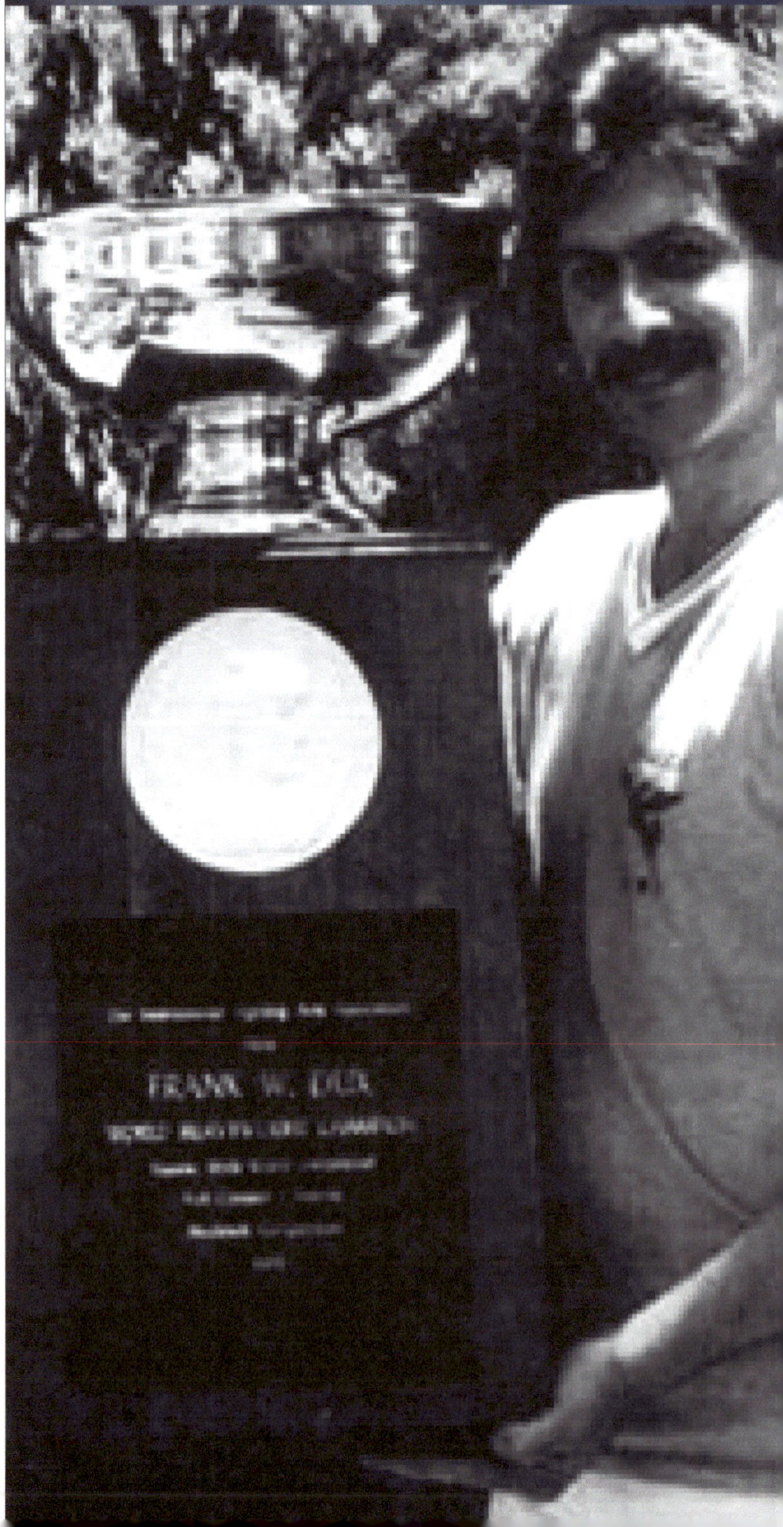

The Gracies may claim dominance, and new champions may rise, but it's the crescendo of Dux's blood-pumping legacy that beats at the heart of combat sports.

As "Bloodsport" burned its images into the retinas of martial arts enthusiasts, it fueled a fire that led to the birth of the Ultimate Fighting Championship. With every punch thrown in the octagon, echoes of Dux's own strikes can be felt.

But the Frank Dux narrative isn't just about fists and feet—it's a saga that stretches into the very soul of martial arts. It is a story not only of a man who achieved unparalleled triumphs but of one who dared to dream of his own fighting league, only to be pigeonholed by the very individuals he wished to elevate.

From the electrifying atmosphere of Paris' Bercy Stadium to the star-studded gatherings in Beverly Hills, Frank Dux moved with the gravitas of a martial arts luminary—his name synonymous with both grandeur and controversy, his legacy a pageant of achievements and unsolved riddles.

Frank Dux remains an enigma—a figure shrouded in legend; his shadow cast long over the MMA world. His journey, a blend of ferocity and finesse, a spectacle of power and resilience, continues to inspire, astonish, and provoke the minds of those who follow in his swift, storied footsteps.

As the curtain falls on the Frank Dux chronicle, one question lingers in the air like the remnant echo of a knockout blow: what is the true measure of a legend, if not the stories that survive the test of time and the roar of the crowd?

For more info visit
www.frankduxbloodsport.com

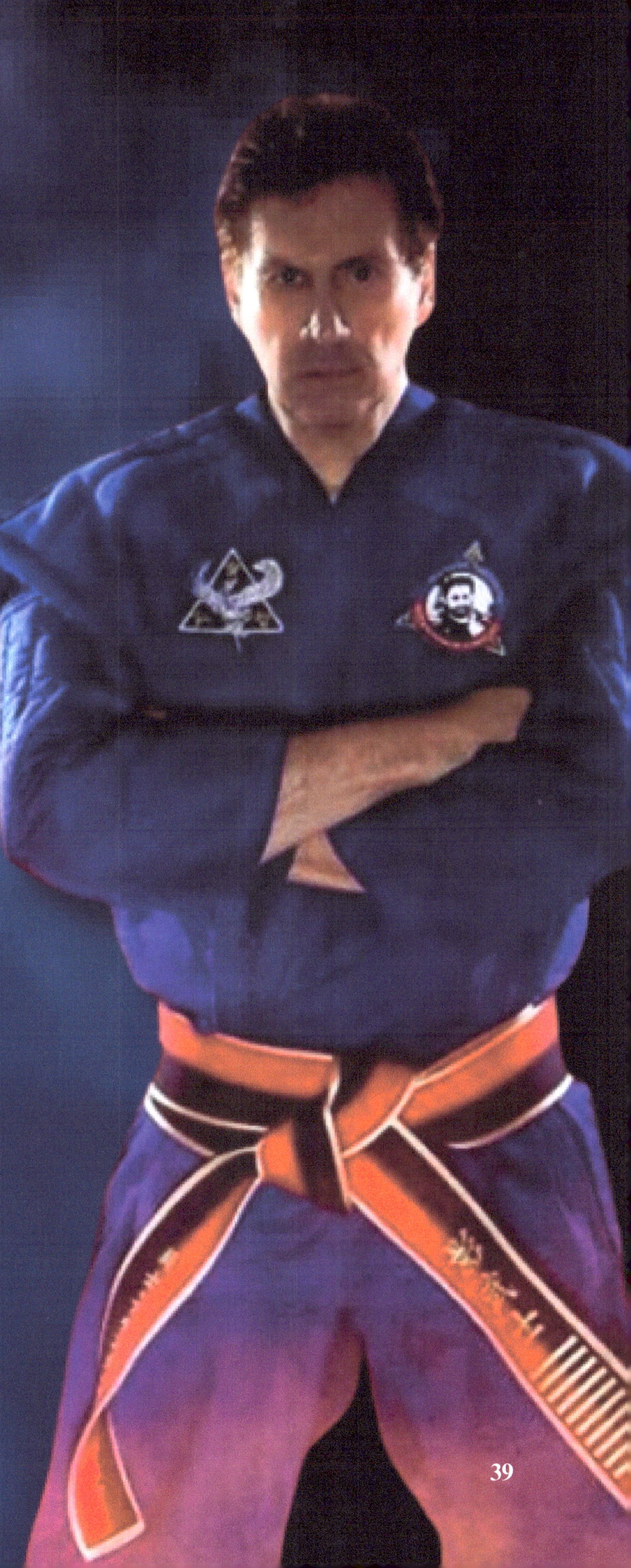

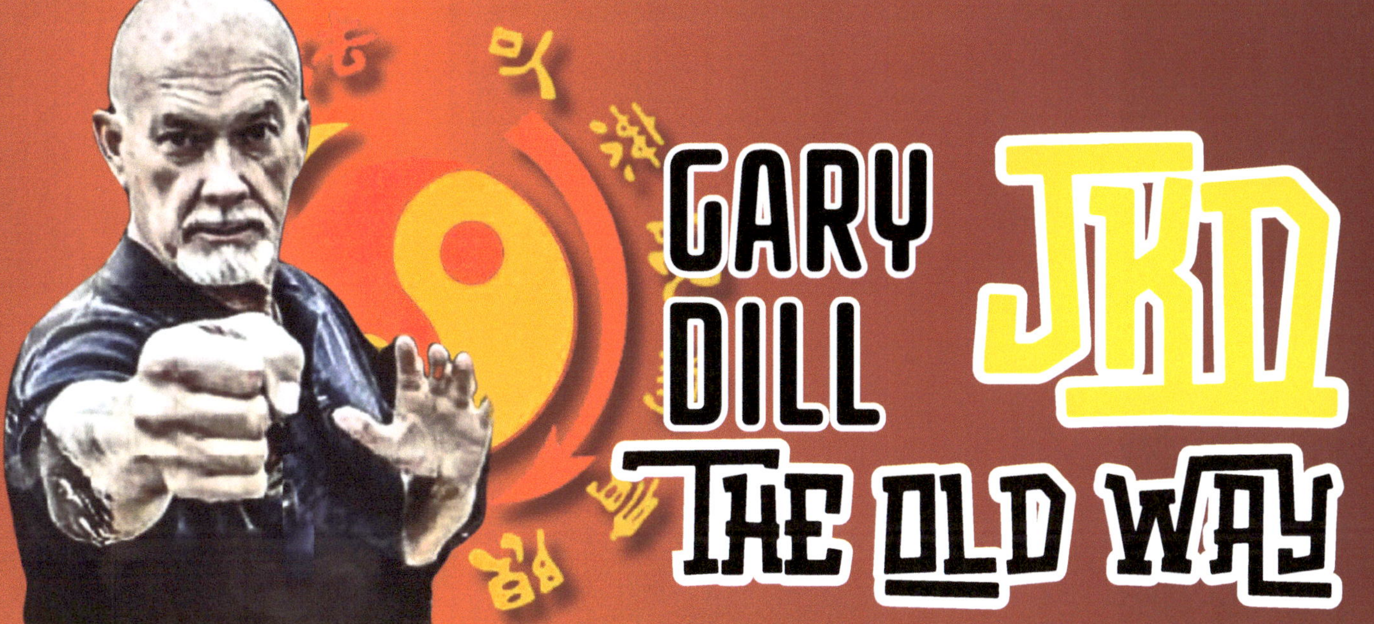

Monthly Column from a true legend in the art. Gary Dill talks about the old ways.

I wrote an article in a 1990 "Inside Kung Fu" magazine in which I introduced the term, "Core Jeet Kune Do" which represents the pre-1973 JKD that Bruce Lee actually developed himself and the way it was taught while he was still alive. The Core JKD is a composite of Wing Chun Gung Fu, Boxing, and Fencing formulated strictly for combat applications (void of sport or aesthetics) which Lee also referred to as "Scientific Streetfighting." This is primarily the focus that I intend to address in future columns.

Who is James Yimm Lee and what was his connection to Bruce Lee and the development of Jeet Kune Do. Of course, Bruce Lee is known all around the world as a martial arts icon. But a name that is not familiar is James Yimm Lee, the gung fu man who had a great influence on Bruce and the development of JKD.

James was one of only three students that Bruce Lee made instructor, with Taky Kimura and Dan Inosanto being the other two. James died just a few months before Bruce which is why there is not much known about him.

Prior to meeting Bruce Lee, James was a well known and highly accomplished Sil Lum kung fu and iron palm instructor in Oakland, California. Having being invited by Bruce in 1962, James, Allen Joe, and George Lee drove to Seattle to meet this young gung fu instructor who was a college student. They were very impressed with Bruce Lee's high skill level in gung fu and they decided to begin what turned out to be years of training under him. Consequently Bruce would drive down to Oakland to give them instructions, and in turn, they would drive to Seattle on a frequent basis for training.

James and Bruce were both no nonsense, dedicated martial artists and they became very good friends. When Bruce married Linda in 1964, they moved to Oakland permanently moving in with James and his family. James was 20 years older than Bruce, but he always considered himself a student of Bruce's. And in turn, Bruce looked upon James as his mentor and surrogate father. James introduced Bruce to body building and hand conditioning (iron palm.)

Because they lived under the same roof, they had the opportunity to train almost every evening together. Bruce used James as his sounding board while experimenting with different techniques in the development of new combat-based techniques. Professor Wally Jay, the founder and grandmaster of Small Circle Jujitsu, lived nearby and was good friends with Bruce and James.

Professor would frequently visit "the garage" during these workouts. He said that Bruce and James would be "extremely rough and would blast each other into the concrete walls of the garage." This was during the Jun Fan Gung Fu period. But after Bruce had the famous fight with Wong Jack Man in Oakland, the workouts became even more intense. Bruce won the fight but felt he could have done better. Even though he spent many years training in Wing Chun in Hong Kong, Bruce felt that in his opinion Wing Chun was lacking in actual combat efficiency and he started to incorporate boxing and western fencing into his fighting system. Thus was the beginning of what we know now as Jeet Kune Do.

Bruce and James had a store front kwoon in Oakland but closed it down because of the overhead expenses. They moved the classes to James Lee garage and that's where they remained until James died in December, 1972. Professor Jay said that It was well known in the bay area that if you wanted to learn JKD you would seek out James Lee and his garage studio. Professor Jay told me that I was lucky to have trained with James instead of Bruce.

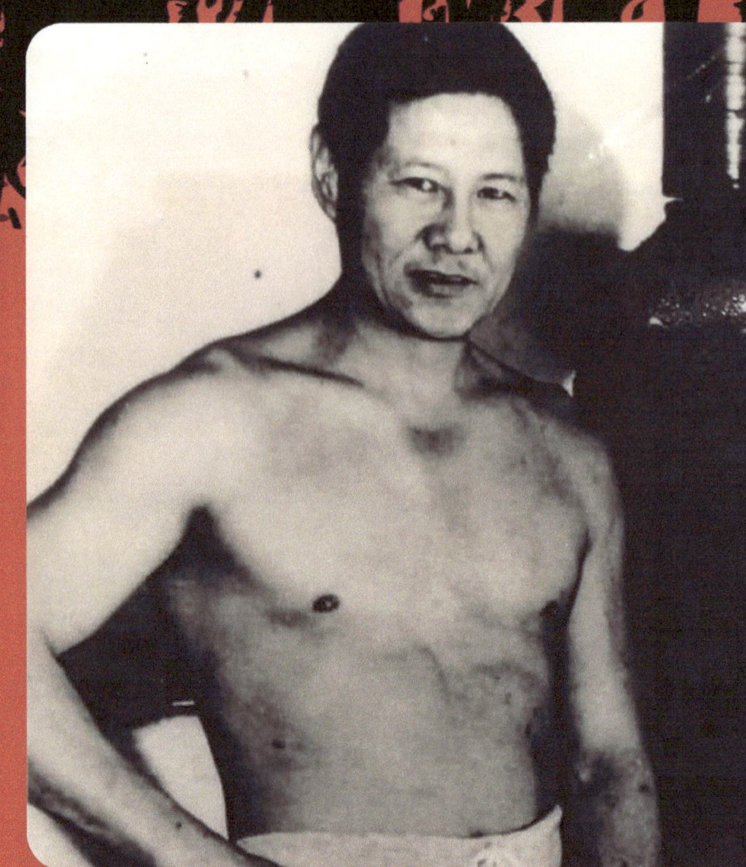

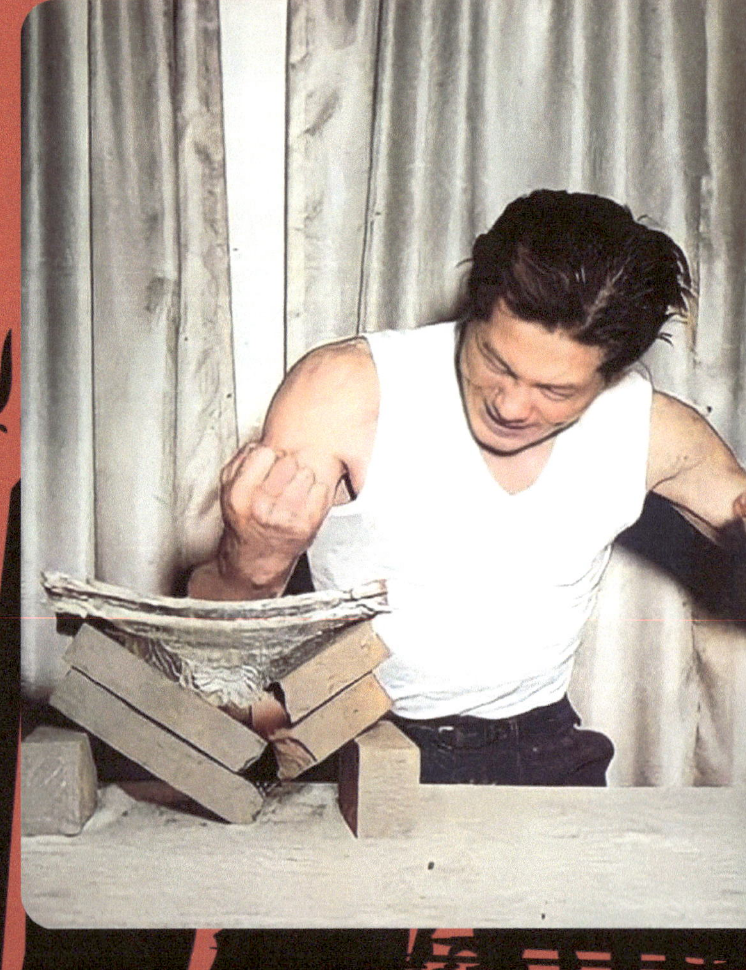

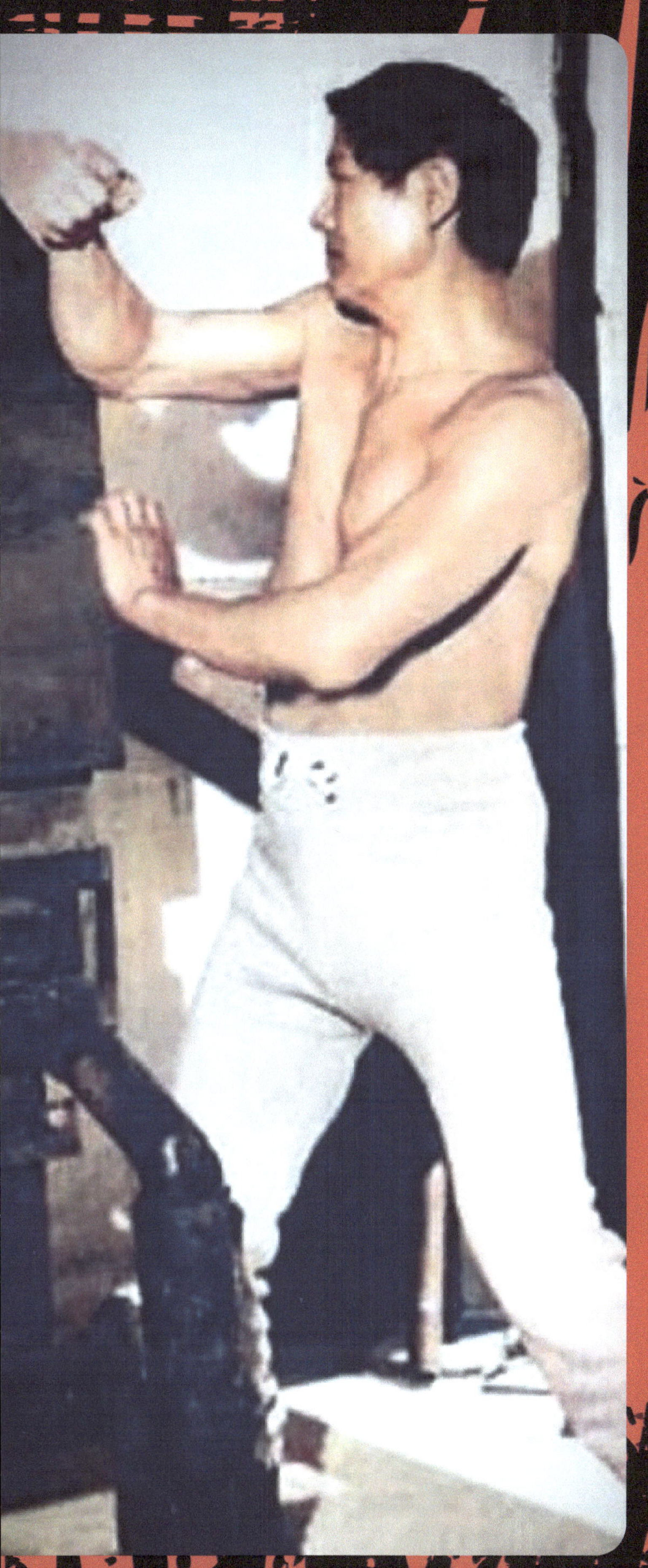

 He said that Bruce was primarily the research and development guy, but James was the teacher and elder of JKD. The Oakland school was known the "JKD Fighting School" because it was so combative in nature.

When Bruce got the job as playing Kato in the "Green Hornet" TV series, he had to relocated from Oakland to Los Angeles. At that time he left James in charge as the primary instructor of the Oakland school. Bruce still was the Oakland Chief Instructor and was responsible for the continuing development of the curriculum. James was very loyal to Bruce and only taught the techniques that Bruce developed and authorized. James was a welder by trade and personally made most of the training equipment that Bruce, he, and the students used. I was accepted as a JKD student in 1971 and was so honored to have trained on the same equipment that Bruce Lee also trained on every day when he lived there, and I worked out in that same garage where JKD was actually developed.

James was a serious instructor with little tolerance and expected 100% effort from students. If someone slacked off, they could not return. During the time I was there I saw him kick out several students. He only wanted students who were serious, open minded, and were dedicated to learn JKD.

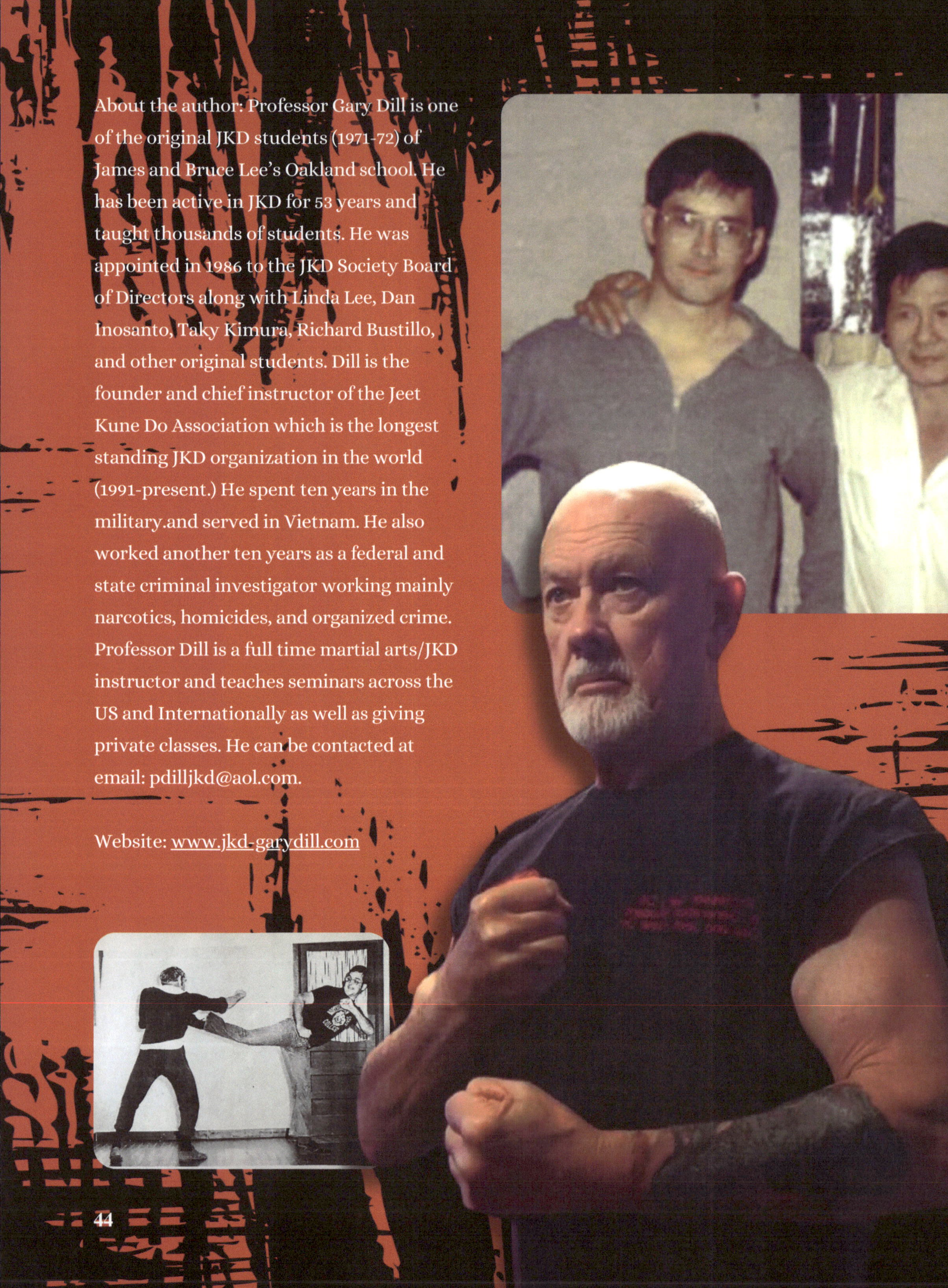

About the author: Professor Gary Dill is one of the original JKD students (1971-72) of James and Bruce Lee's Oakland school. He has been active in JKD for 53 years and taught thousands of students. He was appointed in 1986 to the JKD Society Board of Directors along with Linda Lee, Dan Inosanto, Taky Kimura, Richard Bustillo, and other original students. Dill is the founder and chief instructor of the Jeet Kune Do Association which is the longest standing JKD organization in the world (1991-present.) He spent ten years in the military.and served in Vietnam. He also worked another ten years as a federal and state criminal investigator working mainly narcotics, homicides, and organized crime. Professor Dill is a full time martial arts/JKD instructor and teaches seminars across the US and Internationally as well as giving private classes. He can be contacted at email: pdilljkd@aol.com.

Website: www.jkd-garydill.com

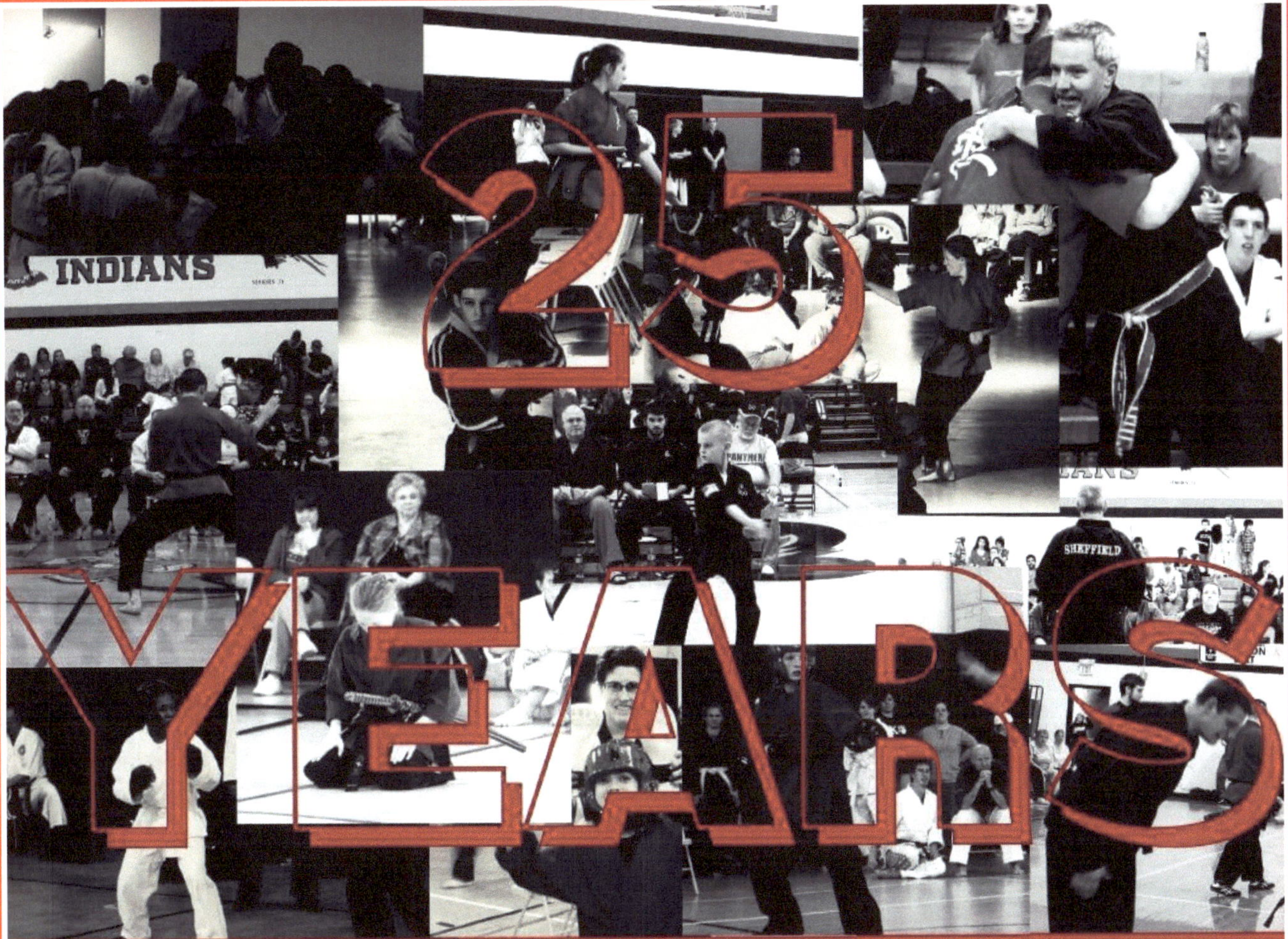

25 YEARS

WARRIOR OF GOD
MARTIAL ARTS CHAMPIONSHIP

SATURDAY, MARCH 9, 2024

616 Cal Young Rd, Hallsville, TX 75650
Hallsville High School

ARE YOU REGISTERED, YET?

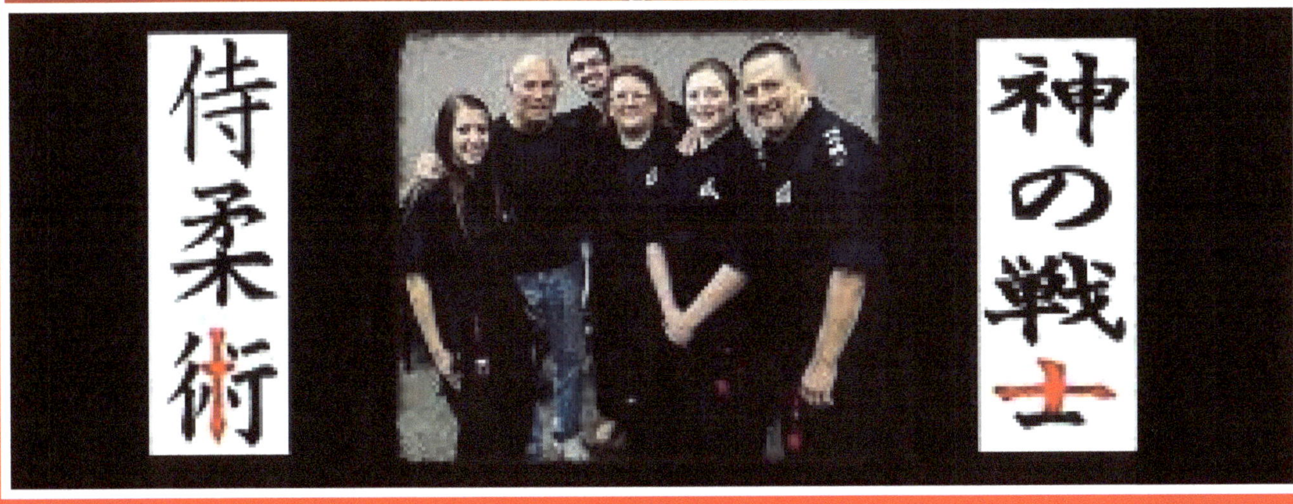

THE KATA

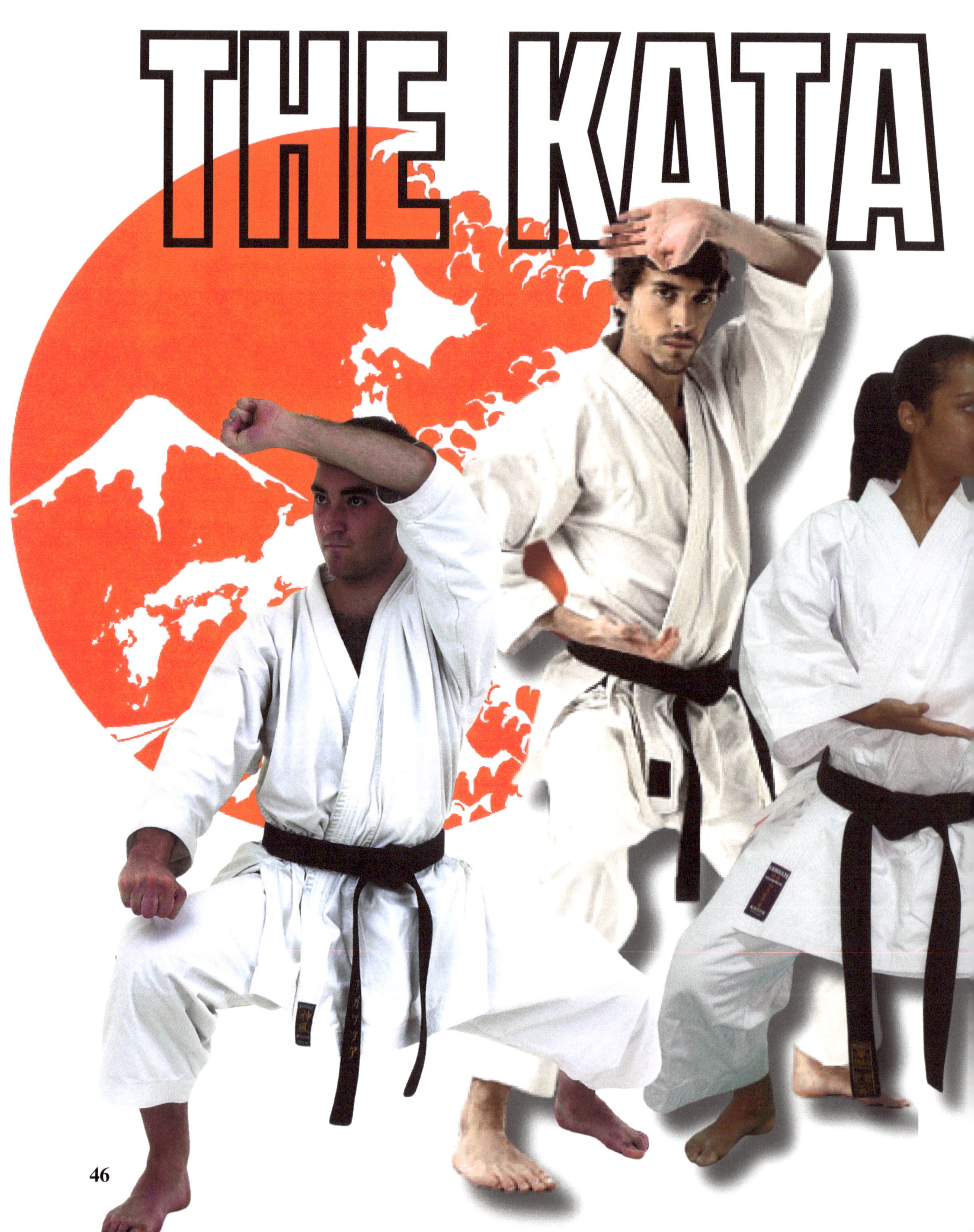

MIND

By Dan Tosh

Most who study karate know that kata is the root and an essential part of the development and pathway to a greater understanding. But what is it that we are trying to understand? Why is kata continuing to be on the lips and in the minds of those who teach and practice karate?

Kata is not only used in martial arts, it is also used in almost everything we do in life that requires learning or repetitive action. A boxer for example does shadow boxing (very much a form of kata). The MMA competitors not only practice with each other, they also work on repetitive movements to instill the auto response required to make the actions become as automatic and reflexive as breathing.

If the need to respond requires time to decide the action in a life-or-death situation, it would be very difficult to make the effective response in the fraction of a second needed to stop the aggression.

 I tell my students that kata is like rehearsing for a play or movie. It not only requires instilled memory, it requires emotion. The emotion of fear, for example, can be a weapon used against you.

To overcome fear requires the practice of mind and body joining in the actions that occur with a visual in the mind that connects the physical and mental state that would naturally occur in a heated moment of survival against a predator.

Movement without an emotional and meaningful connection has no lasting result. If the kata is done properly, it will reveal the weaknesses as well as the strengths in the actions taken in the movements, we call kata. Those weaknesses can be minimized, and the strengths can be enhanced by the proper performance of kata.

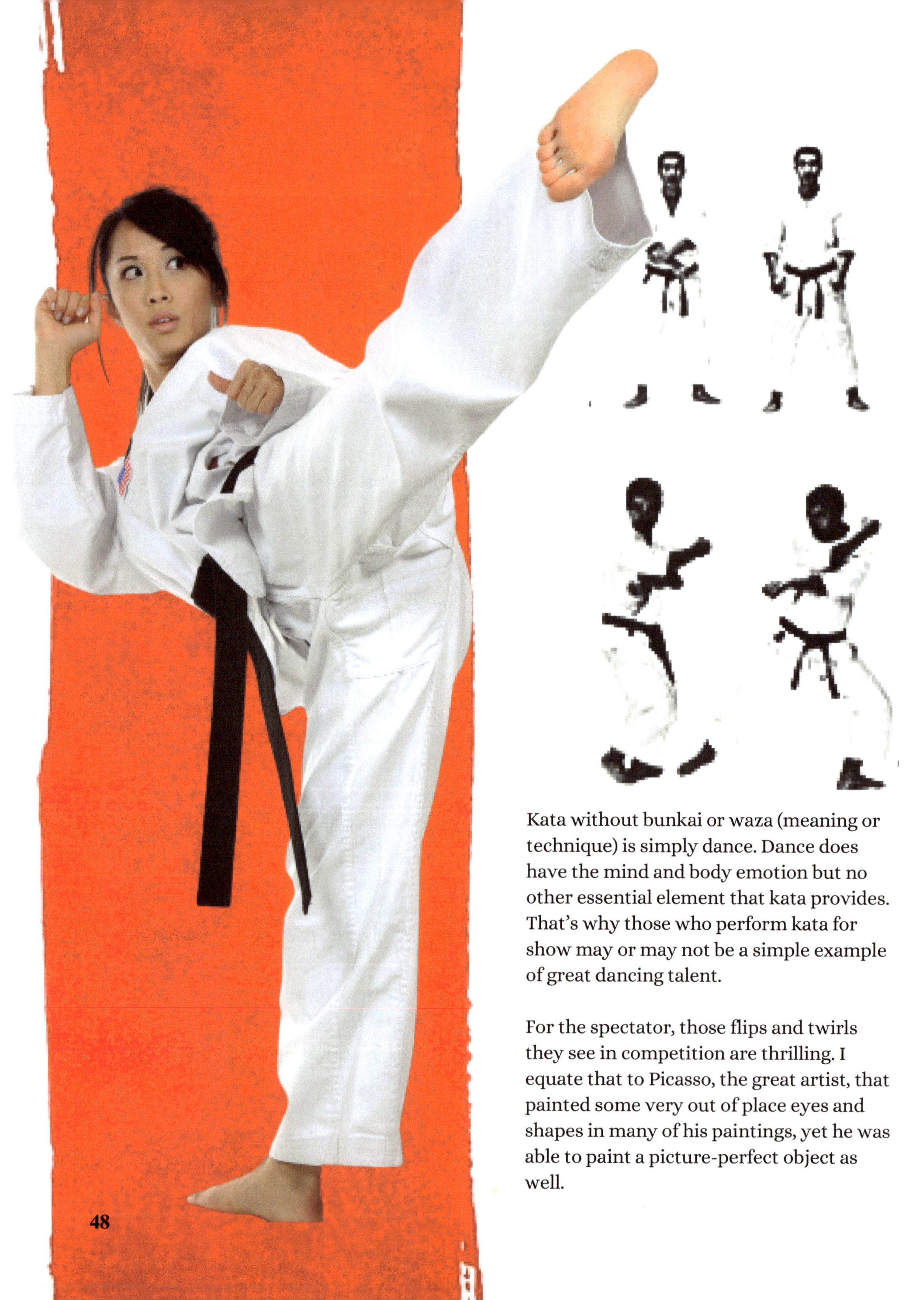

Kata without bunkai or waza (meaning or technique) is simply dance. Dance does have the mind and body emotion but no other essential element that kata provides. That's why those who perform kata for show may or may not be a simple example of great dancing talent.

For the spectator, those flips and twirls they see in competition are thrilling. I equate that to Picasso, the great artist, that painted some very out of place eyes and shapes in many of his paintings, yet he was able to paint a picture-perfect object as well.

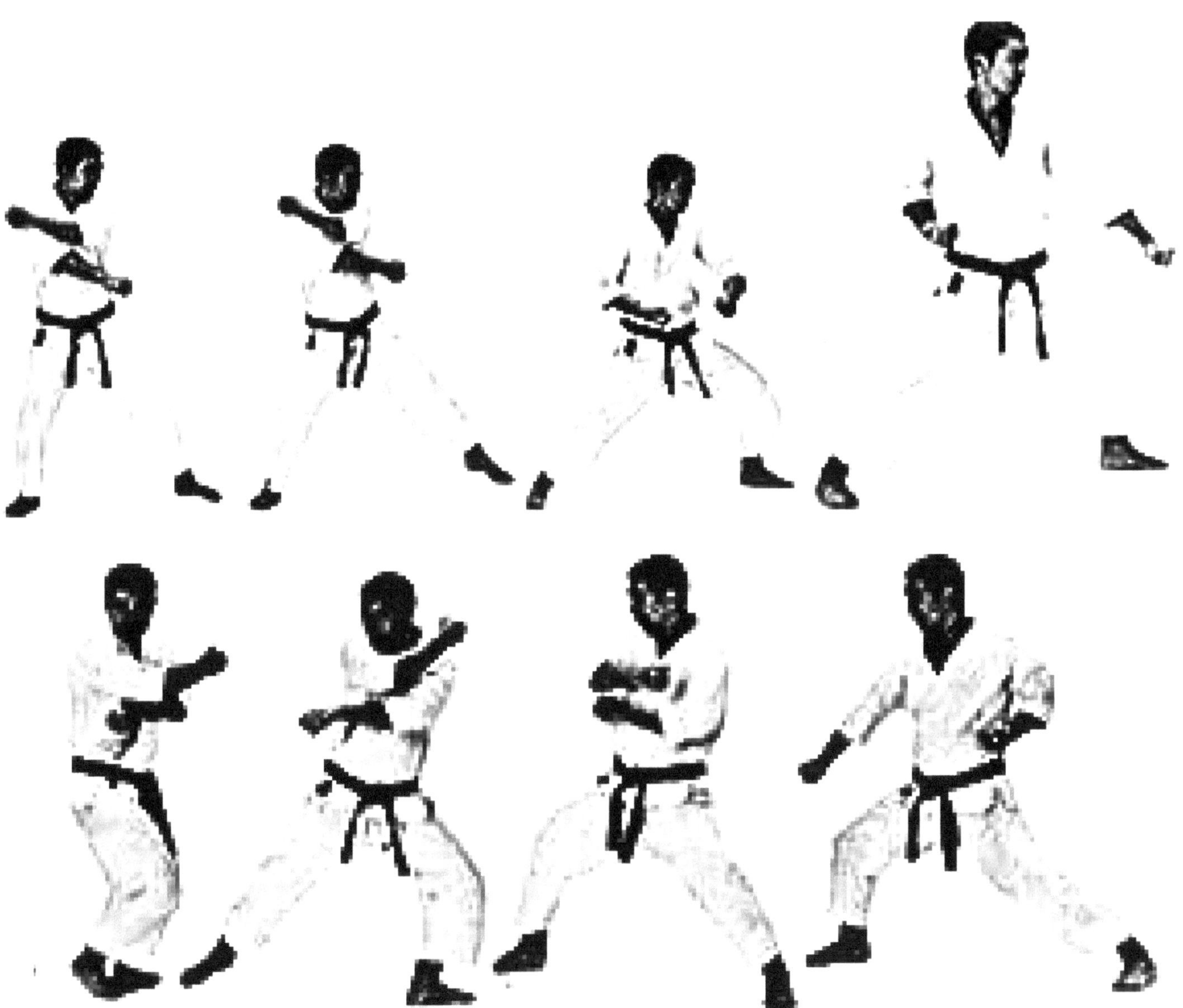

Those who create empty minded kata, that also know the beauty and meaning of a kata that represents an effective action or reaction to the would-be opponent are truly gifted.

If kata is done with the correct mindset, the beginning includes a rei, dei, or bow. That movement is not for respect, although it certainly could be, it is for the transition from the calm and safe place you are to the dangerous place that you can see in your mind, the place that requires action to thwart off the attacks that are coming.

The next movements require an immersive mind and body relationship. The actions that take place now are very real. When you do this repeatedly, you slowly gain the auto-response required for any attack that corresponds with the attack.

The unexpected additional benefit of kata is that not only does each movement have meaning, but all the movements in every kata that you practice can be combined with any movement from any other kata. This gives you an endless number of reactions to literally any attack that could ever take place.

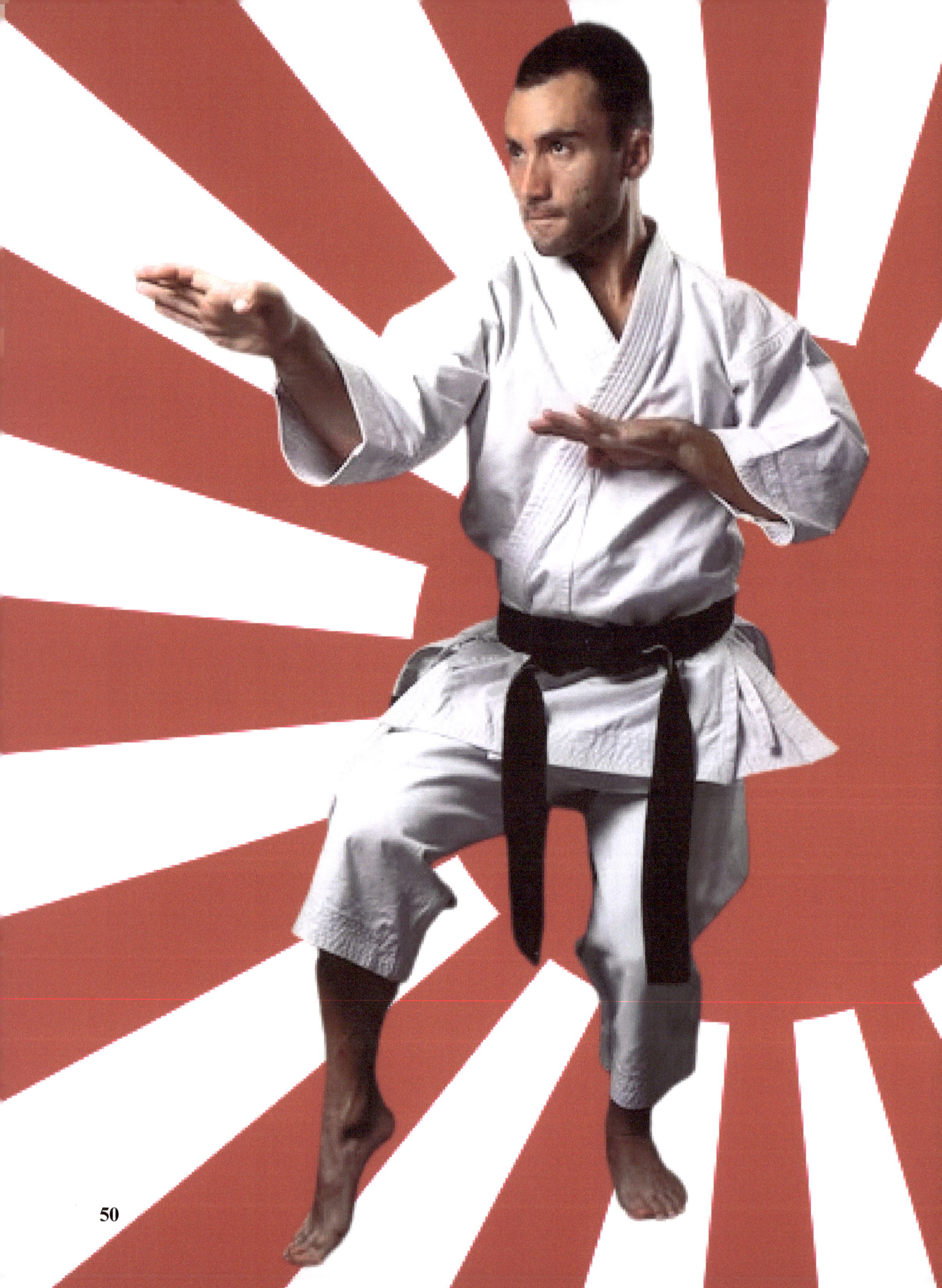

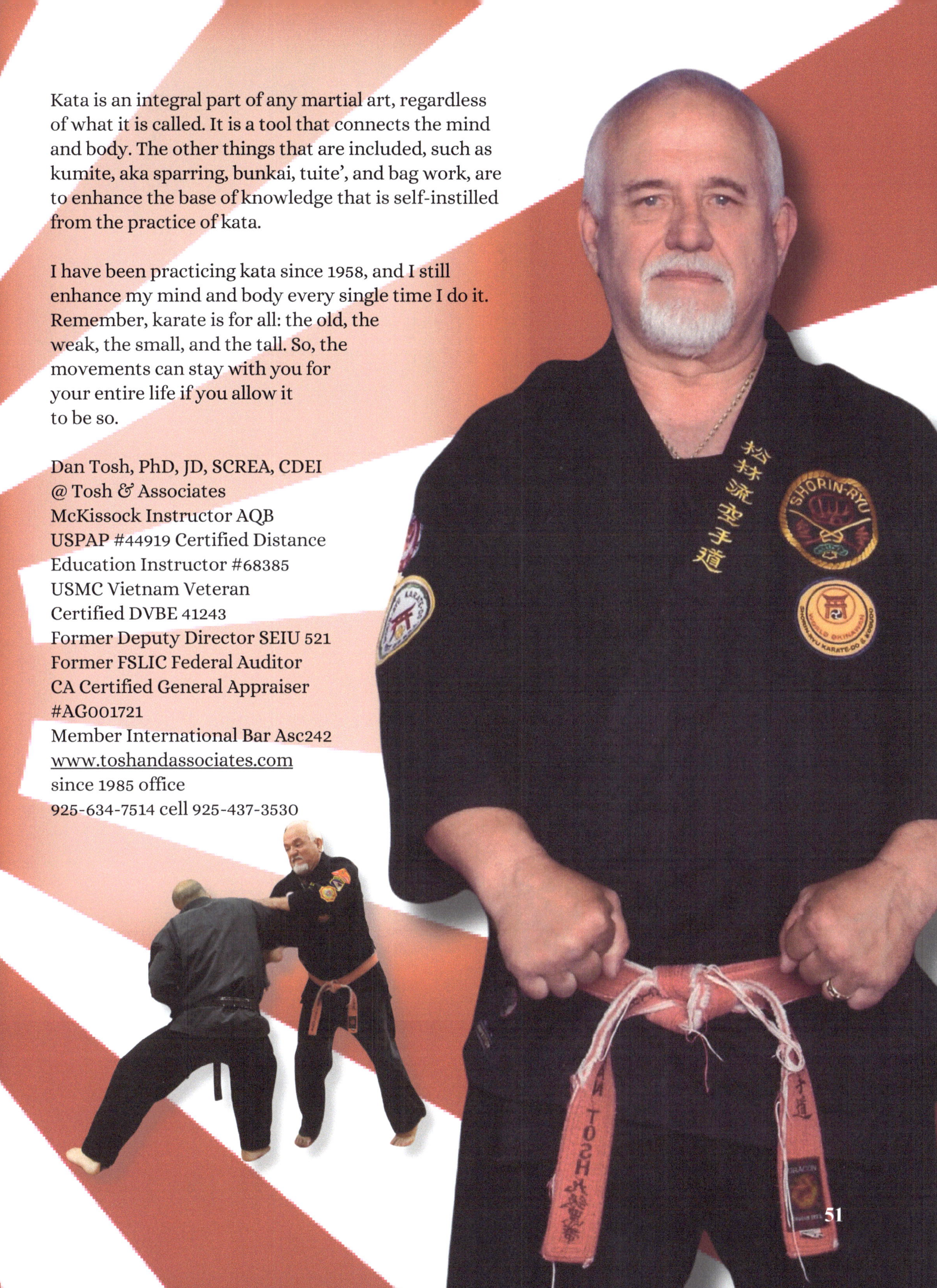

Kata is an integral part of any martial art, regardless of what it is called. It is a tool that connects the mind and body. The other things that are included, such as kumite, aka sparring, bunkai, tuite', and bag work, are to enhance the base of knowledge that is self-instilled from the practice of kata.

I have been practicing kata since 1958, and I still enhance my mind and body every single time I do it. Remember, karate is for all: the old, the weak, the small, and the tall. So, the movements can stay with you for your entire life if you allow it to be so.

Dan Tosh, PhD, JD, SCREA, CDEI
@ Tosh & Associates
McKissock Instructor AQB
USPAP #44919 Certified Distance
Education Instructor #68385
USMC Vietnam Veteran
Certified DVBE 41243
Former Deputy Director SEIU 521
Former FSLIC Federal Auditor
CA Certified General Appraiser
#AG001721
Member International Bar Asc242
www.toshandassociates.com
since 1985 office
925-634-7514 cell 925-437-3530

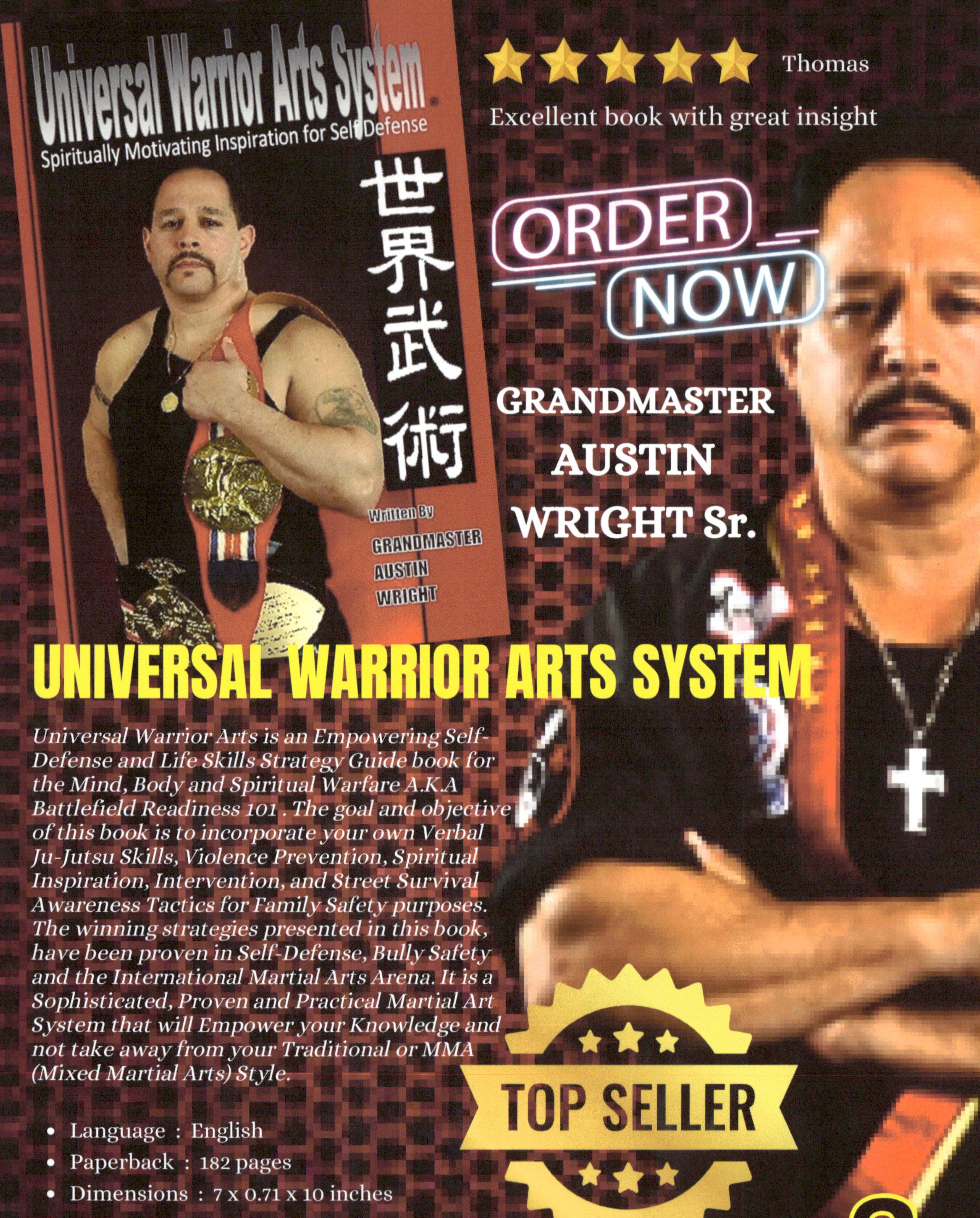
Universal Warrior Arts System
Spiritually Motivating Inspiration for Self Defense
世界武術
Written By
GRANDMASTER
AUSTIN
WRIGHT
Thomas
Excellent book with great insight
ORDER
NOW
GRANDMASTER
AUSTIN
WRIGHT Sr.
UNIVERSAL WARRIOR ARTS SYSTEM
Universal Warrior Arts is an Empowering Self-Defense and Life Skills Strategy Guide book for the Mind, Body and Spiritual Warfare A.K.A Battlefield Readiness 101 . The goal and objective of this book is to incorporate your own Verbal Ju-Jutsu Skills, Violence Prevention, Spiritual Inspiration, Intervention, and Street Survival Awareness Tactics for Family Safety purposes. The winning strategies presented in this book, have been proven in Self-Defense, Bully Safety and the International Martial Arts Arena. It is a Sophisticated, Proven and Practical Martial Art System that will Empower your Knowledge and not take away from your Traditional or MMA (Mixed Martial Arts) Style.
• Language : English
• Paperback : 182 pages
• Dimensions : 7 x 0.71 x 10 inches
TOP SELLER
AVAILABLE ON AMAZON.COM

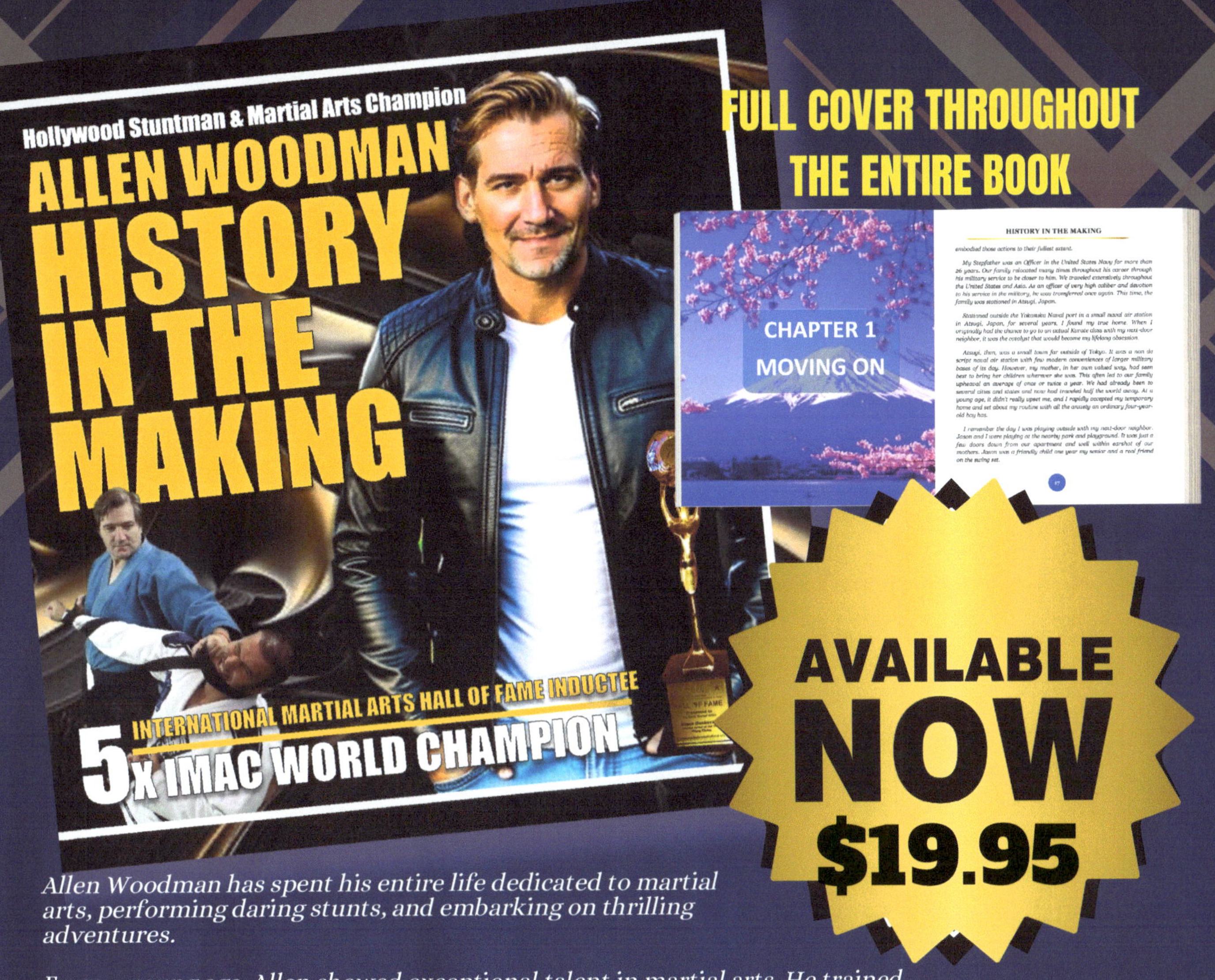

Allen Woodman has spent his entire life dedicated to martial arts, performing daring stunts, and embarking on thrilling adventures.

From a young age, Allen showed exceptional talent in martial arts. He trained tirelessly, honing his skills and becoming a champion in various disciplines. His passion for adventure led him to travel to different countries, immersing himself in different cultures and learning from the best martial artists around the world. But Allen's story isn't just about martial arts.

With a keen business mind. He successfully established several businesses in different countries, making a name for himself as an entrepreneur. His ability to adapt to new environments and connect with people from different backgrounds played a crucial role in his success.

Throughout his journey, Allen encountered numerous challenges and obstacles. But he faced them with determination and a positive outlook. His wit and perspective on life makes him a captivating storyteller, sharing his incredible journey with the world. In his book, Allen recounts his 50 years of life experiences. His unique perspective on life, adventure, and business made his story a captivating read for anyone seeking inspiration and excitement.

His story serves as a reminder that with dedication, resilience, and a positive mindset, anyone can overcome challenges and create a life filled with adventure, success, and fulfillment. If you're looking for a captivating story that combines martial arts, adventure, and business, Allen Woodman's book is a must-read. Prepare to be inspired, entertained, and motivated.

$4.95 FULL COLOR DIGITAL VERSION ONLINE WWW.ISSUU.COM

AVAILABLE ON AMAZON.COM

IMAC TOURNAMENT

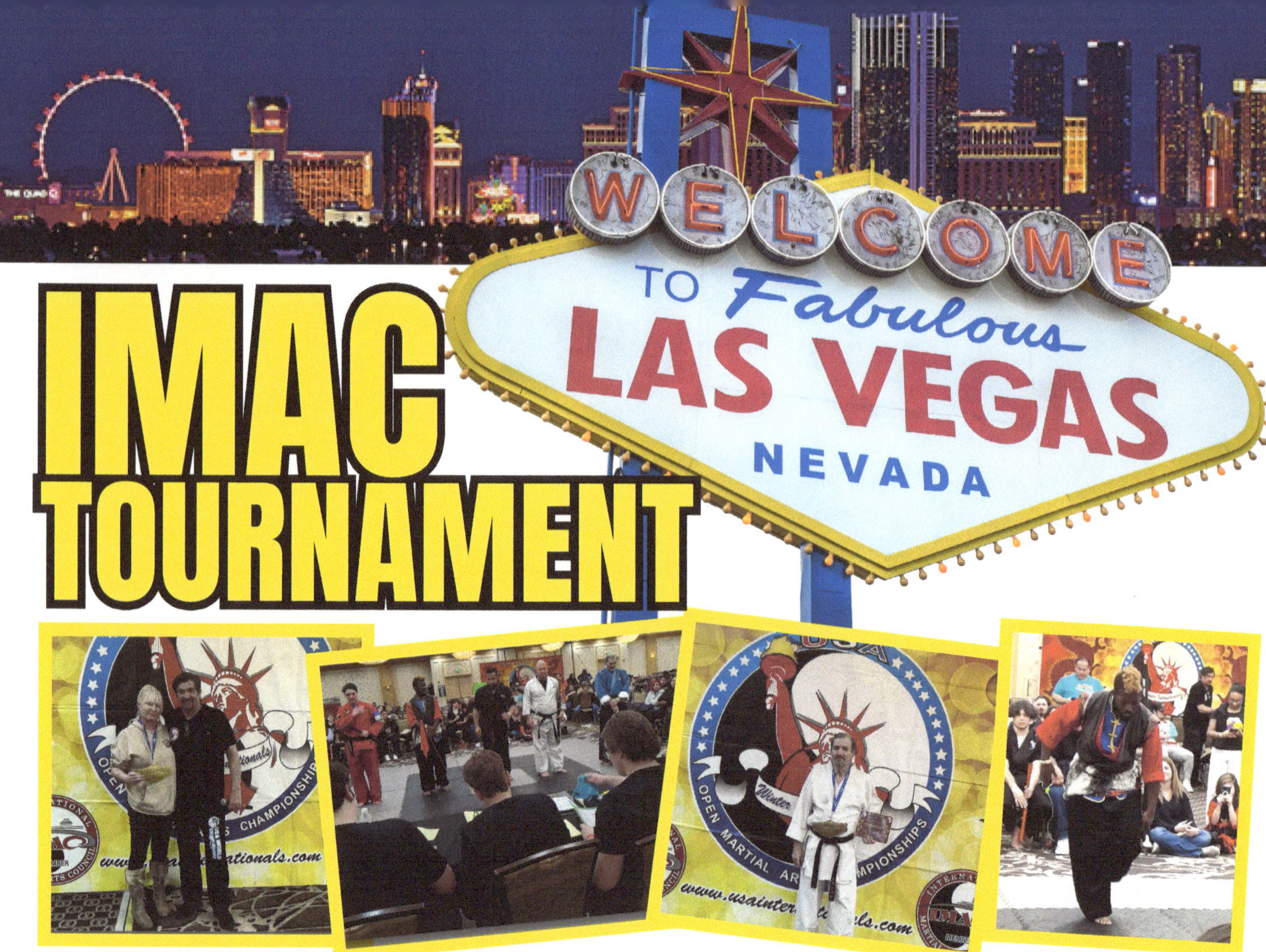

The IMAC International Open Karate Championship in Las Vegas, the city of neon lights, played host to a spectacular display of martial arts talent on February 3, 2024.

The one-day event, the IMAC International Open Karate Championship, was a convergence of skill, discipline, and competitive spirit, bringing together participants from across the United States, Mexico, and Canada. Promoted and hosted by Stan Witz, the tournament lived up to its reputation for excellence. The event has become a staple in the martial arts community, known for drawing amazing talent and pitting competitors against each other at the peak of their game.

All the competitors were vying for the coveted title of World Champion.

The tournament showcased an array of categories, including forms, weapons, and fighting, with each participant demonstrating their hard-earned expertise. Impressively, the event was conducted without a single instance of injury or impolite behavior, a testament to the discipline and respect ingrained in the martial arts culture.

Spectators were in for a treat, not only from the high-level competition but also from the presence of a few celebrities.

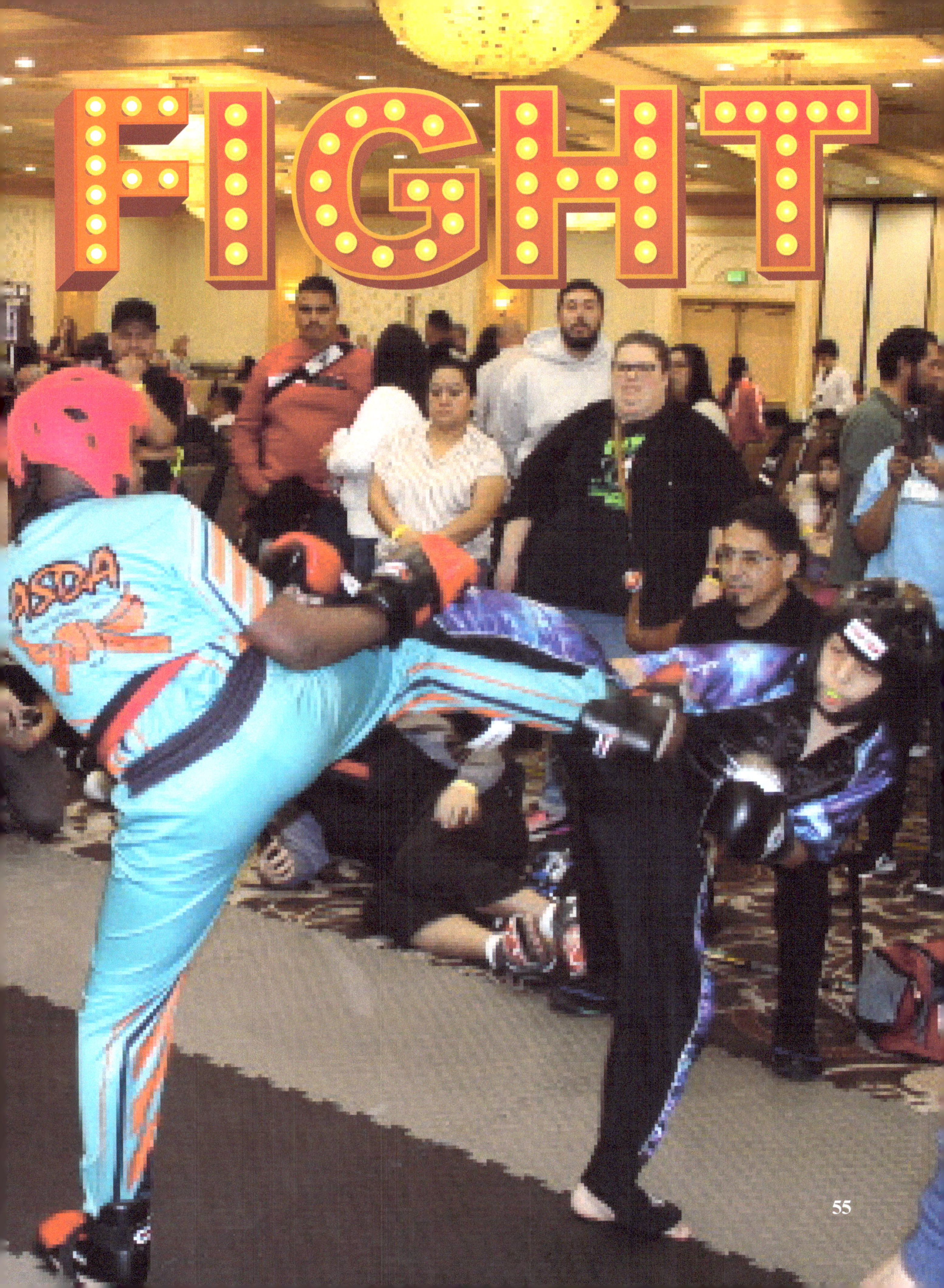
FIGHT

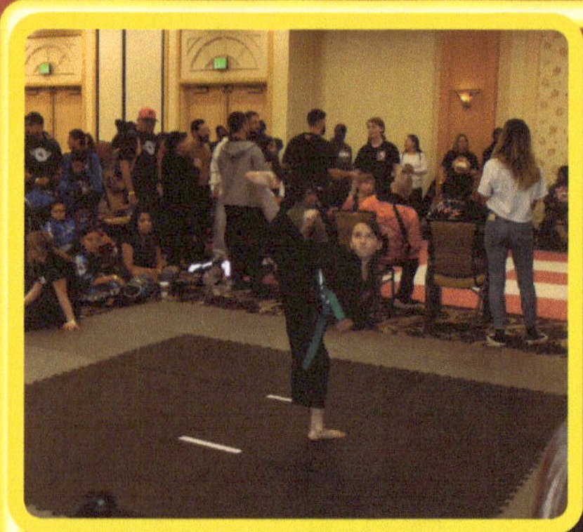
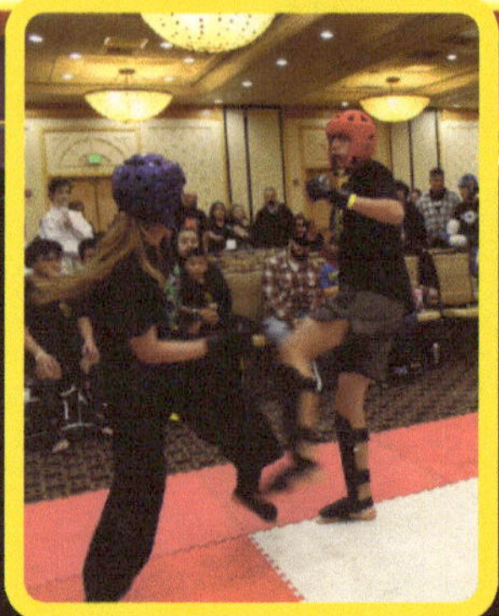
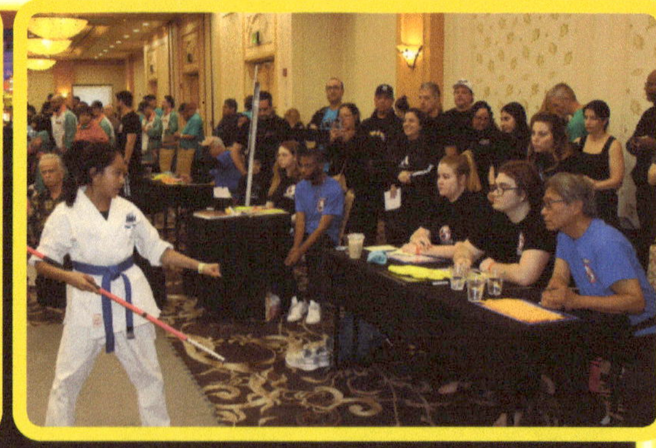
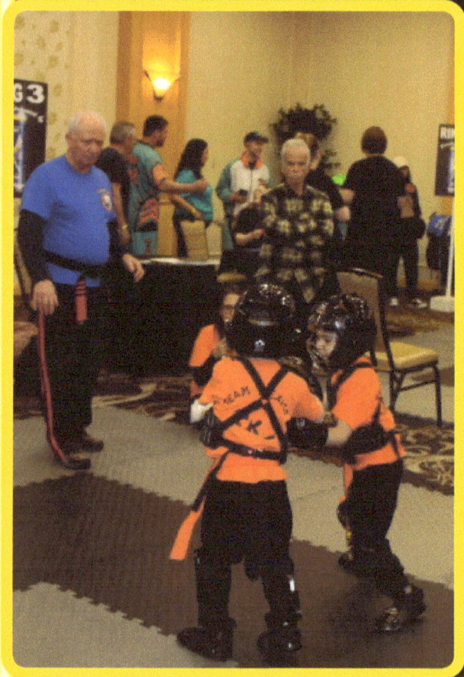
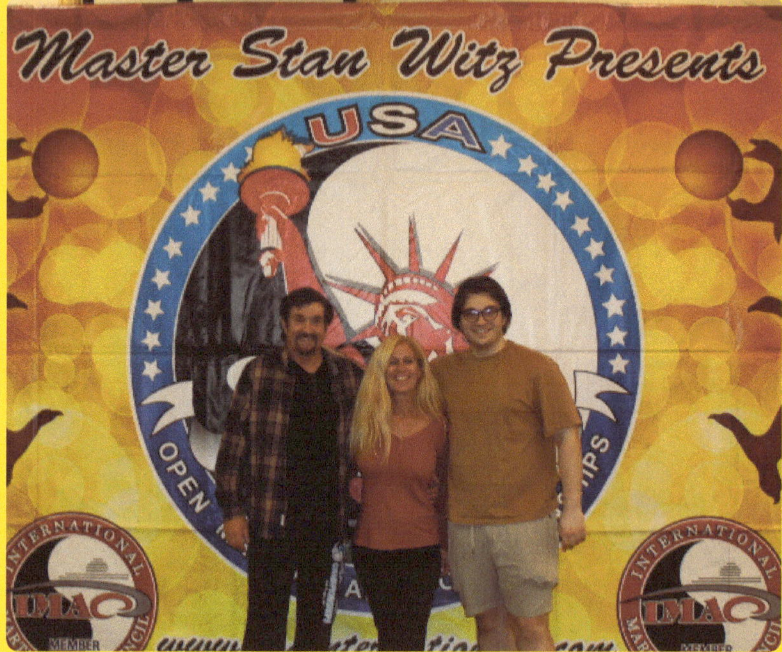

Master Stan Witz Presents
USA
OPEN
INTERNATIONAL
IMAC
MEMBER
INTERNATIONAL
IMAC
MEMBER

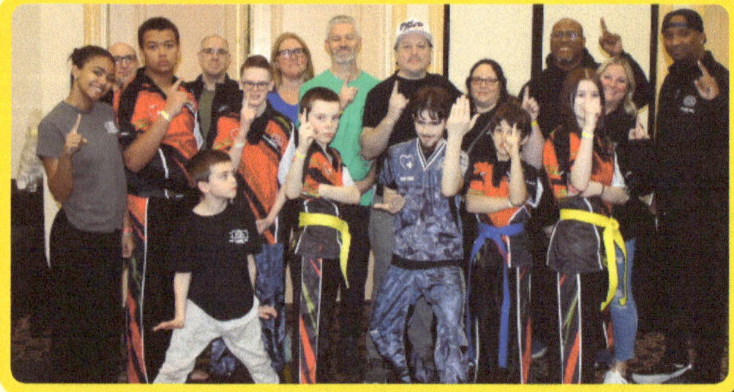
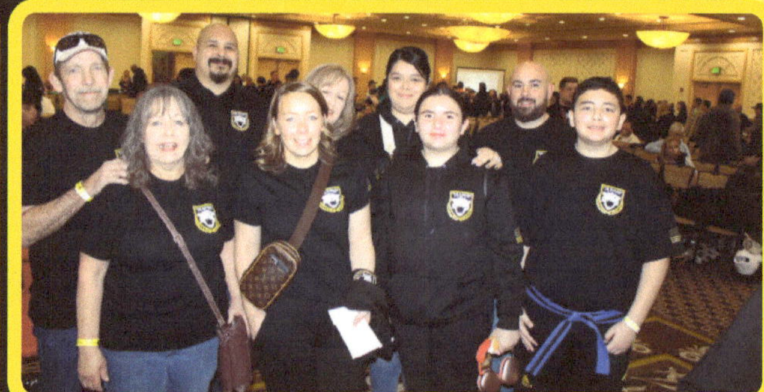
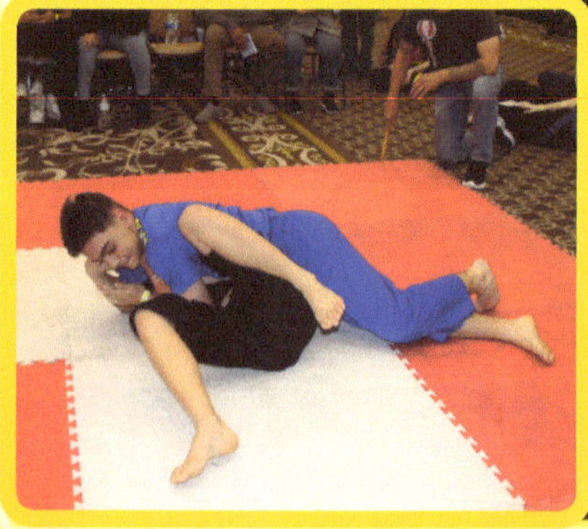
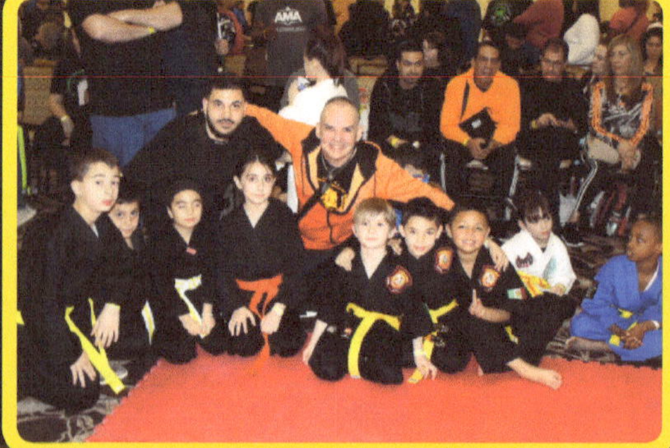
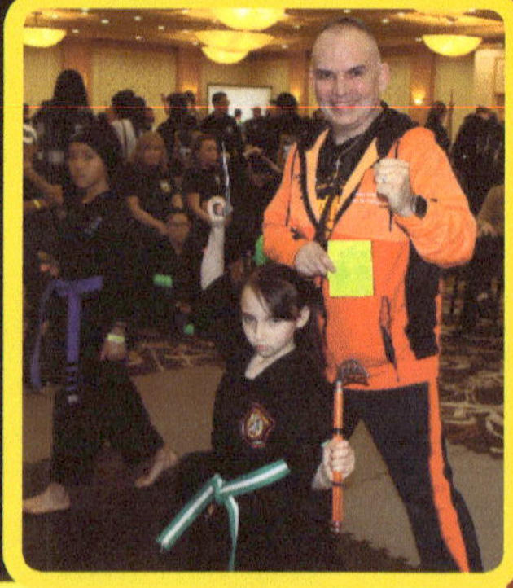

IMAC CHAMPIONS
BLACK BELT DIVISION

SELF DEFENSE

Brynlee Krehbiel
Ethan Blain
Kate Alk
Laurelle Blain
Madison Franzen
Madison Kitterman
Mitch Shimer
Paul Casey

BREAKING

Lonnie Walker
Abbigal Veis
Bob Houghton
Brynlee Krehiel
Lexilee Veis

GRAPPELING
Grappling - No Gi

Everest Slawinski
Fujiko Slawinski
Gabriel Novak
Isabella Rodriguez
Michael Lennox

CONTROLLED SPORT MMA

Acelyn Reilly Kirk
Elly Chavez
Isabella Rodriguez
Jade Chavez
Leo Santiago
Michael Lennox

KICKBOXING

Abbigael Veis
Everest Slawinski
Fujiko Slawinski
Guillermo Montanaro
Isabella Rodriguez
Jerry Cazales
Mathew Montepio
Mia Serrato
Michael Lennox
Black Belts

EXTREME WEAPONS

Musical Weapons
America Cox
Briselle Garibaldi
Jessica Carson
Lonnie Walker
MC Harshaw

CREATIVE WEAPONS

America Cox
Briselle Garibaldi
Kloris Bronson
Laurie Healy
Lonnie Walker
Lonnie Walker
Madisyn Franzen
MC Harshaw
Sara Bronson

TRADITIONAL WEAPONS

Briselle Garibaldi
Jace Dawley
MC Harshaw
Oliver Carson
Sara Bronson
Tammy Wight

MUSICAL FORMS

Briselle Garibaldi
Lonnie Walker

CREATIVE FORMS

Briselle Garibaldi
MC Harshaw
Damen Caballero

JAPANESE FORMS

Briselle Garibaldi
MC Harshaw
Dalton Grove

CHINESE FORMS

Jimmy Wight
Madison Hobbs
Oliver Carson
Sean Lawrence

TKD FORMS

Cage Young
George Fullerton

KENPO FORMS

America Cox
Briselle Garibaldi
Kekoa Perbera
Kloris Bronson
Laurie Healy
Madisyn Franzen
Paul Casey
Sara Bronson

POINT SPARRING

America Cox
Angelo Key
Briselle Garibaldi
Elijah Elliot
Jace Dawley

FORMS

James Engler
Jerry Cazales
Kekoa Perbera
Laurie Healey
Madisyn Franzen
Mathew Montepio
Michael Engler
Rusteen Salehi
Zerek Fulbright

WEST COAST

America Cox
Jerry Cazales
Laurie Healey
Mathew Montepio
Zerek Fulbright

More information available on www.**usaworldchampionships.com/imac-champions**

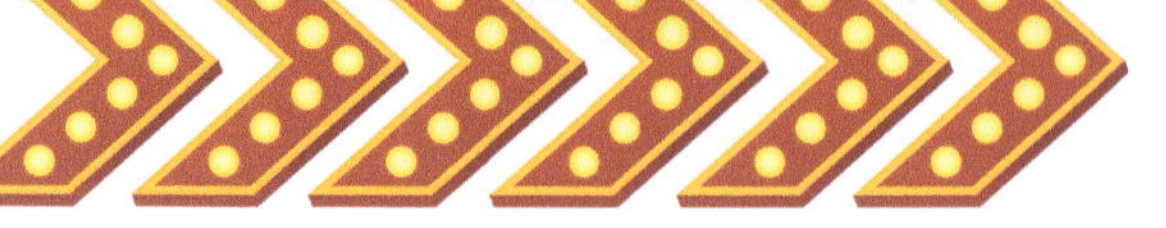

Martial arts legends like Peter 'Sugarfoot' Cunningham and Allen Woodman graced the event, supporting their students and friends, adding a touch of star quality to the already exciting proceedings. Notable among the winners was Mitch Shimer who clinched the intermediate Self Defense Category.

Allen Woodman made a commendable third-place finish in the traditional weapons division, while MC Harshaw showcased versatility by placing in various divisions, including weapons, forms, and fighting. The crowning moment came with the announcement of the world champion in the fighting division, marking a grand finale to the event.

The combination of fair judging and excellent directing contributed to the smooth execution of the tournament, closing it on a high note and setting the stage for success in subsequent events. As participants and enthusiasts reflect on the triumphs and memories of the February event, they can look forward with anticipation to the next gathering of martial arts talent, already scheduled for June 2024.

In a city that never sleeps and constantly dazzles, the IMAC International Open Karate Championship stands out as a beacon of martial arts excellence, leaving us all waiting eagerly for the next chapter in this ongoing legacy of world-class competition.

Stay tuned for the next IMAC International Open Karate Championship set for June 2024. For more information and updates.

Keep up with martial arts icons like Peter Cunningham and Allen Woodman by following their social media pages for insights, tips, and motivational content.

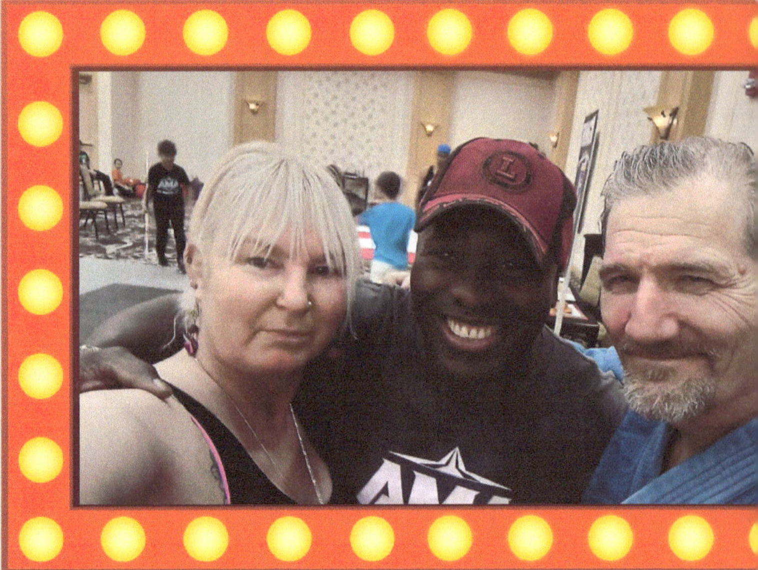

IMAC Champions Mitch Shimer, Peter Sugarfoot Cunningham and Allen Woodman Enjoying the great day of fights, forms, and weapons at the IMAC Championships in Las Vegas, Nevada.

REAL SELF DEFENSE FOR WOMEN

Joseph J. Truncale ★★★★★
A fantastic book filled with practical tips

Keith McCarary ★★★★★
Unveiling the Harsh Reality of Abuse and Equipping Women with Effective Self-Defense
.

Women in today's society are often the target of crime and personal attacks.Societal perceptions of the weaker sex make women a target for those who would use their size, weight or aggression against another person. With information gleamed from the most renown Law Enforcement agencies around the world, this book covers the perception of sexual assaults and the statistics from around the globe to tell a stunning and often horrific storyline about abuse and women's issues in today's society. Real Self defense that is useful and easy to learn with step by step directions.

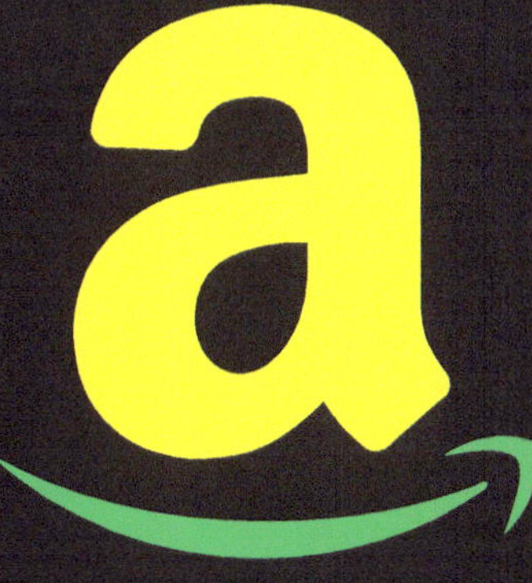

293 pages
Language
English
2019
Dimensions
7 x 0.66 x 10 inch

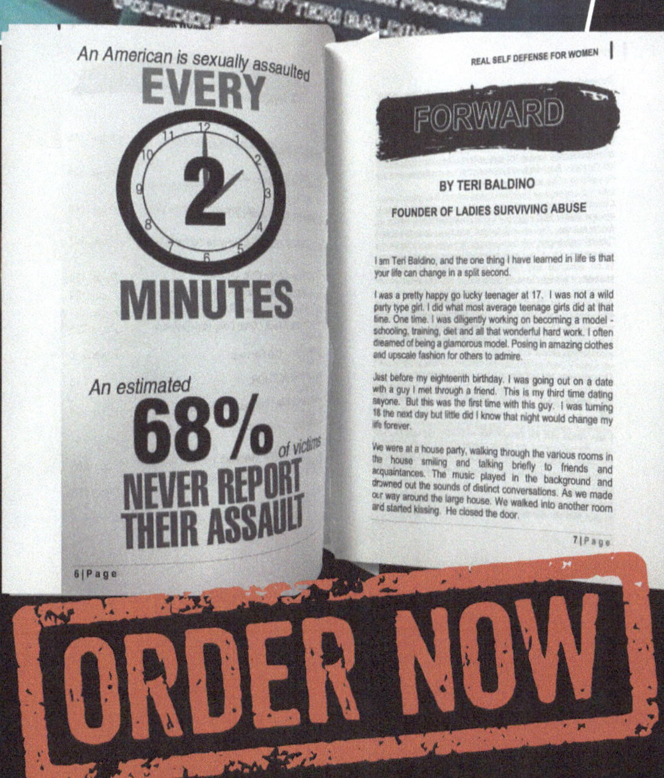

ORDER NOW

$11.95
+ S & H

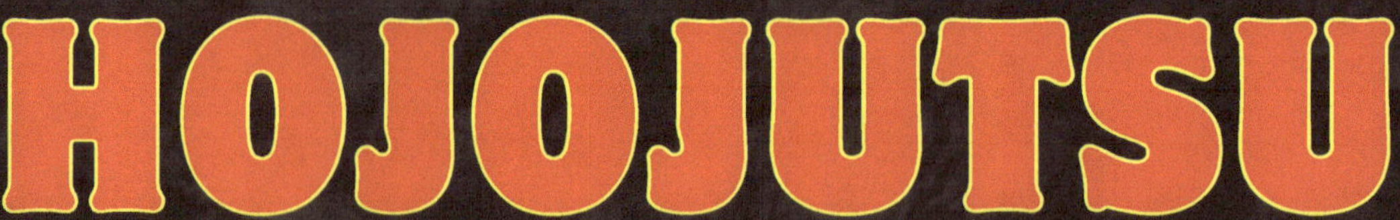

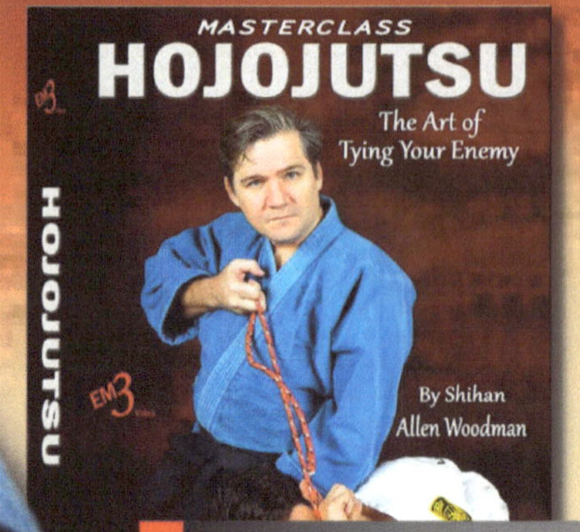

HOJOJUTSU
The Art of Tying Your Enemy
DVD 1
47 bmin.

$14.95
+ S & H

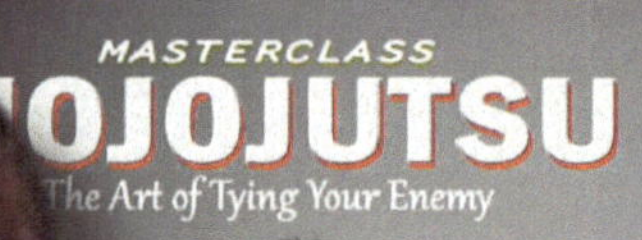

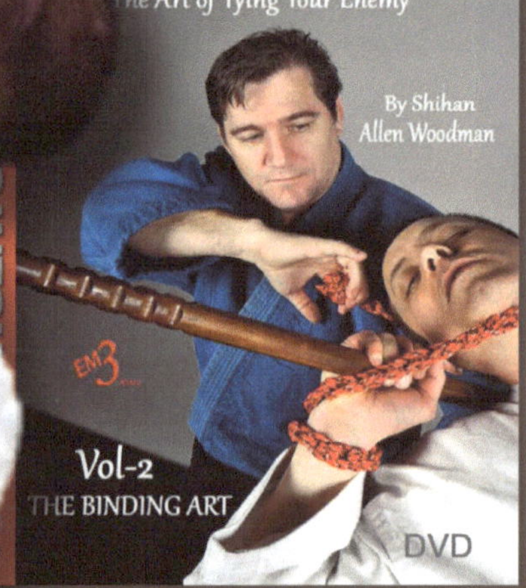

★★★★★
HOJOJUTSU
The Art of Tying Your
Enemy
DVD 2
49 bmin.

$14.95
+ S & H

★★★★★

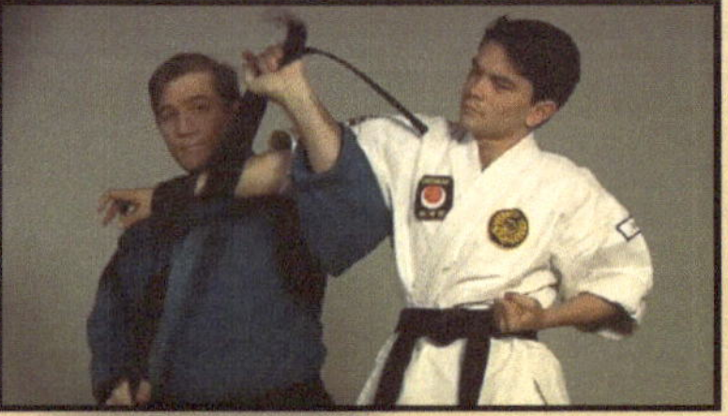

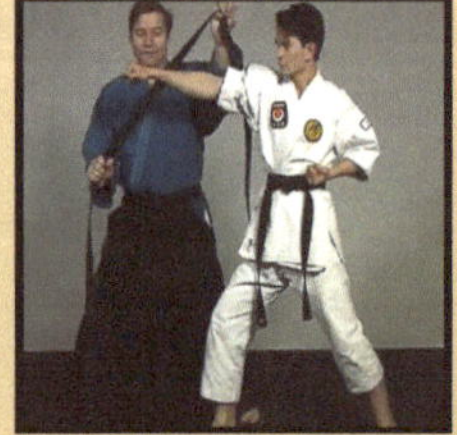

Step-By-Step Instruction throughout full color video

ORDER NOW

AVAILABLE ON AMAZON.COM

Available for workshops / Seminars / Events / Book Signings

BOOKS & DVD

Hojojutsu is a traditional Japanese martial art of restraining that encompasses different school techniques. It is a unique product of Japanese history and culture and is rarely practiced outside Japan. It is part of the curriculum under the aegis of bugei and in jujutsu. There are very few videos or books available on this art. Shihan Allen Woodman teaches you hands-on each technique in a step-by-step format.

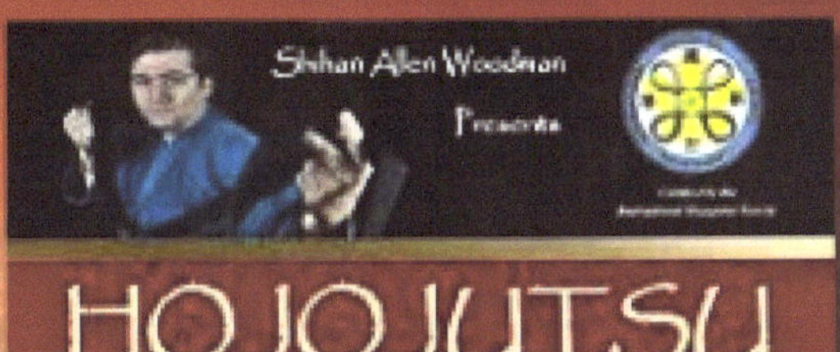

VOL 1 / VOL 2 $29.95 +S & H

FULL COLOR INTERIOR DIMENSIONS 8X8 132 Pages

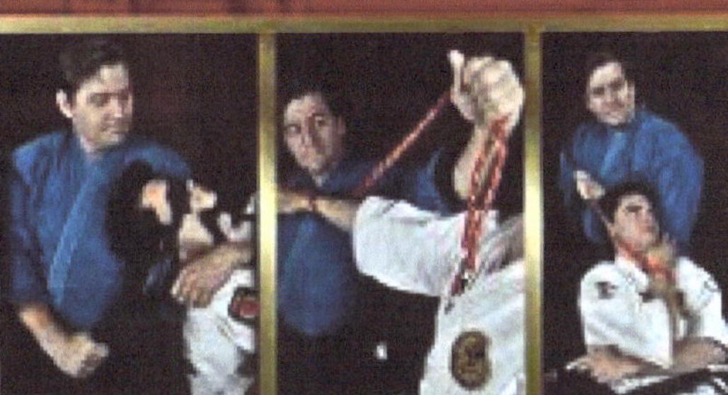

★★★★★

Good information to add to what is presented in class.

★★★★★

New concept, for America, really effective

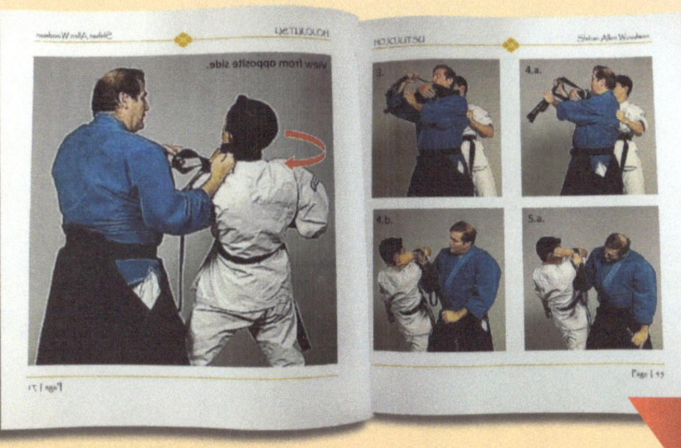

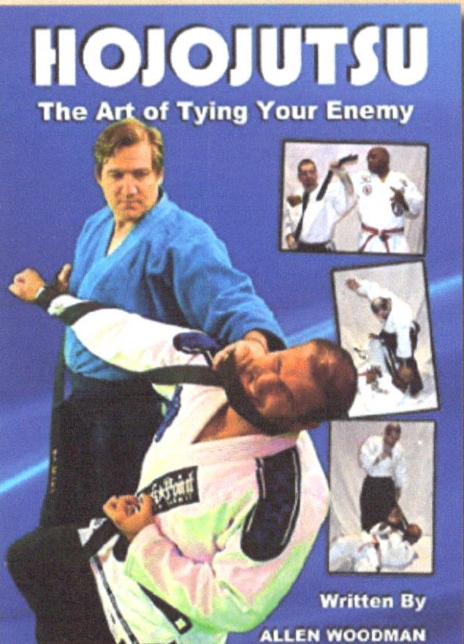

$9.95 +S & H

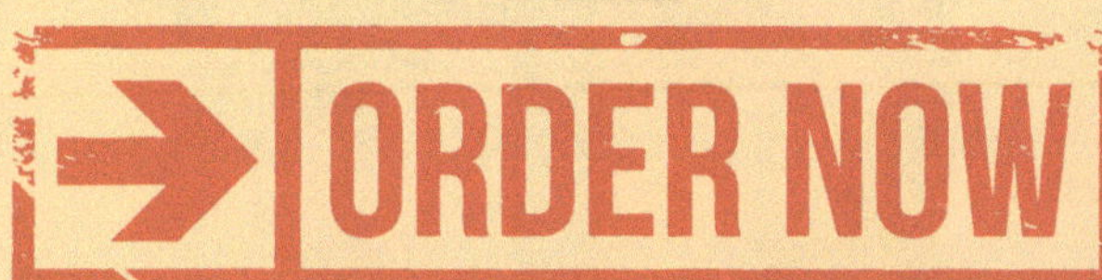

→ ORDER NOW

1 (725) 377-8092

allenwoodman1967@gmail.com

AVAILABLE ON AMAZON.COM

Available for workshops / Seminars / Events / Book Signings

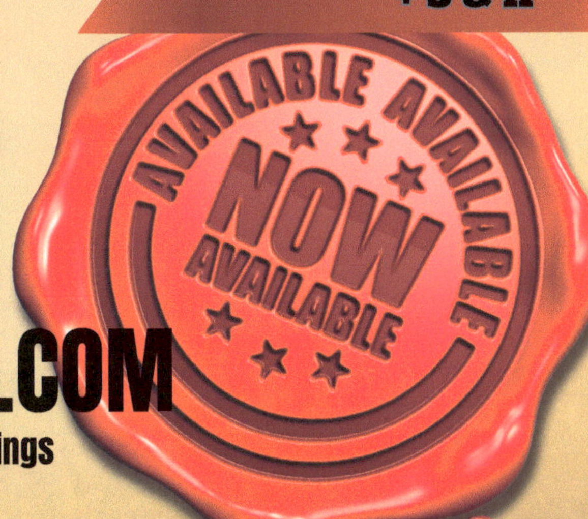

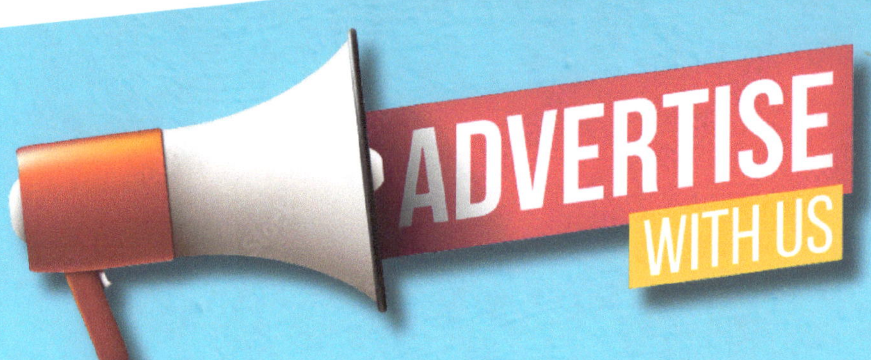

Would you like to be featured in our magazine? Do you have a product you would like to promte? Would you like your event advertised in our magazine? Contact us to learn how.

FULL Page
Full Color

$150

Back Cover
Full Color

$250

1/2
Half Page
Full Color

$75

Large Discounts for multiple issue advertising

1/2
Half Page
Full Color

$65

1/4
Page
Full Color
$25

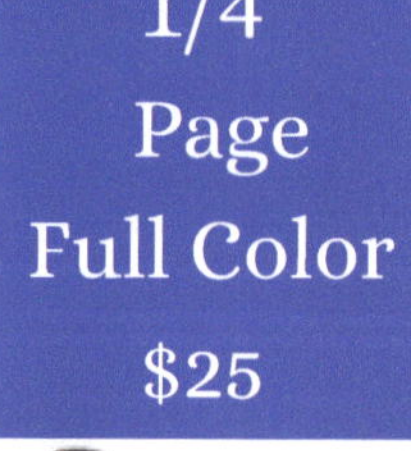

1/3
Page
Full Color

$45

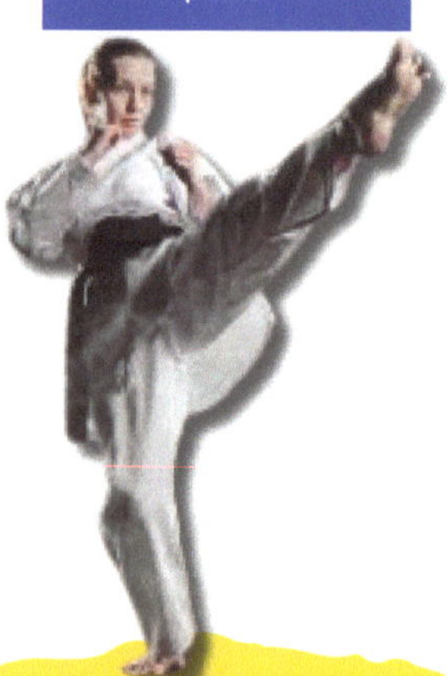

artseastpublish@gmail.com /
www.internationalmamagazine.com
1 (725) 377 - 8092